WHC [illegible]

KEY LESS[illegible] F ADULT CHILDREN RETURNING TO LIVE AT HOME

MINIMIZING CONFLICTS AND MAXIMIZING OPPORTUNITIES TO STRENGTHEN FAMILY BONDS

VICTORIA LYNCH

To my adult children who I love beyond measure.
Thank you for sharing your life's journey with me.

CONTENTS

INTRODUCTION

Isn't life interesting? As parents, we raise our children to be independent and know someday they will leave home to pursue their dreams. We all will experience mixed emotions of sadness and pride simultaneously when they finally leave their childhood home and find we may have to make some adjustments to our own lives when this happens.

Adapting to the processing of the change you are going through, or the *mourning period* of them leaving home, never to live with you again, could even be taking place around the same time they approach you to move back in with you. Or perhaps it has been some time since they have lived at home, and you have settled into a new rhythm at home. You might even be thinking about the possibilities of grandchildren on the horizon, or maybe they are here already, and you are enjoying this new experience. Whatever stage you find yourself at in your life, when your adult child approaches you to move back home, the relationship you are experiencing with them now may change.

How do you deal with this? Some may think this is an easy process as they are your children after all, aren't they?

In this new phase of your life and now having to navigate those twists and turns of having your child back at home can be an exciting and enjoyable time, but it is very different from what you both know. Be mindful of the effect and the potential it may have in disrupting the cozy nest you have developed with your spouse without the children at home. Your patterns of behavior, your schedule of activities, and the flow of your daily routine without considering anyone else but yourselves will be a few of the important things in your current life that will have some sort of shift.

Recognizing that this burgeoning phenomenon is becoming more common, and realizing that you are not alone in this experience of mixed emotions that will surface, is the first acknowledgment to be made to yourselves as parents. It even has a name —*boomerang children/kids*—which is quite apt to describe adult children needing to return home after living independently, but due to various circumstances they need to move back home.

This book explores the steps you can take to create a peaceful home environment with clear boundaries for each other's needs and expectations when your adult child returns to live at home. It is also specifically aimed at tackling issues of these adults returning to the nest for a defined period to attain a specific goal. Long-term multi-generational living or living with elderly parents is not covered. However, some aspects of this book may be applicable in these situations.

This book also does not address whether or not you should allow your adult children to move back home. Everyone's circumstances are different, and it would be a personal evaluation of your situation if you decide it is a yes, or a no.

SO, WHAT COMES NEXT?

Everyone wants to avoid conflict, especially at home—your safe place, your nest, and a place to have no judgment where you can just be yourself. Maintaining peace and sanity at home comes with an understanding of the enlightenment of how negative feelings affect everyone in the household. The necessity of finding strategies that work right from the beginning of this new time of living together again will help avoid potential conflict that could surface when it comes to identifying and clarifying each other's boundaries. It is also an opportunity to have easy and open conversations about each other's boundaries that will create a good balance between the adult and child, as this has now evolved into an adult-to-adult relationship.

And then, allowing yourself to discover the awareness and the importance of the dynamics that will surface that could ultimately change your relationship will stand you in good stead!

No matter what your home, emotional and financial situations are, when your adult child approaches you about moving back home, it will create an upsurge in some feelings. These feelings could be angst, joy, uncertainty, or relief, just to name a few, but also more than likely will be a combination of all of these and more. Everyone's situations are different, and aspects from financial stability to physical spaces will need careful consideration. The most critical point is to maintain clear communication regarding the expectations of the parent(s) and the adult child. This should be discussed before they move back in; for example, how long they intend to stay and what the motivating factor may be for them to have decided and requested to come and live back home.

Statistics for the number of adult children returning to live with their parents are rather interesting. Two questions that pop up regularly are:

1. What are the reasons for adults moving back home?
2. Are they staying forever, or is it just for some time to get themselves back on their feet?

It seems that the main reason is financial, but it can also range from emotional upheavals (such as divorce) or a tragedy (such as the death of a partner/child/friend) to global world crises. The cost of living has increased exponentially, and it is not uncommon for people to share homes these days to attempt to reduce the exorbitant cost of living that pressures everyone. Adult children moving back home for a period is becoming more the norm than the unusual.

Taking three countries, the United Kingdom, the United States of America, and Australia, and focusing on the age group between 20 and 30 years presented some interesting results. The findings are listed below for your interest.

- The United Kingdom

A whopping 3.5 million adult children live at home with their parents. This number is a combination of those who have never moved out or returned home. This number has increased by a third in the past 10 years. Loughborough research has indicated that 71% of adult children continue to live at home until their early 20s. Adults between the ages of 25 and 34 who own their own houses have fallen from 55% in 1996 to 34% in 2016 (Hayes, 2022). In 2021, adult children living at home grew to 42% (Clark, 2022).

- The United States of America

From February through to May 2020, the number of adult children between 18 and 29 years who lived at home with their parents rose from 47% to 52% in a relatively short time. The most recent data compiled in October 2021 brings the figure down slightly to 46% (Wagner, 2021).

Most recent research by the Federal Reserve Bank of Cleveland indicates that most adult children that move back home stem from the higher-income bracket of families. Families that earn over $140,000 annually show that 36% have adult children returning home, whereas only 10% are from families that bring in less than $27,000 (Hess, 2022).

- Australia

More than 50% of adults live with their parents throughout Australia (Conversation, 2020). In a survey conducted in 2020 with just over 1,000 Australians, it was recorded that 34% of households had adult children. However, in follow-up research that was done post-lockdown regulations stemming from the pandemic, 43% of these adult children in this group have subsequently moved out (Dastoor, 2021).

This reality of adult children moving back home is a growing trend; perhaps the empty nest syndrome may be moving towards a thing of the past. An undeniable contributing factor was the effect of the COVID-19 pandemic, which had a significant impact on the number of families moving in together. The economic and social implications placed upon our world due to this pandemic may be long-term. One sure thing is that you are not alone. This book will also provide insight into helping you navigate this journey that can sometimes be challenging.

WHY YOU SHOULD READ THIS BOOK

As a parent, if you are asking yourself any of the questions listed below, then you should read this book. As an adult moving back home, this book is just as important for you to read to gain some perspective of what your parents will be encountering and understand their feelings to help create a positive input. It is a book with helpful information and guidance, plus some resource material that can help everyone in this new journey together. It is also an opportunity to gain some wisdom and advice from others in the same situation. Consider these questions:

- What should I be aware of if my adult children come back to live at home for a period of time?
- What strategies should I implement to avoid conflict and mixed emotions that may surface?
- What steps should I take to deal with this shift in our relationship, whether short-term or long-term?
- How do I create and enforce the boundaries for a healthy and new adult–adult relationship?

Who Stole My Fish?

You might be wondering why this is the title of the book. It seemed the perfect choice to bring my own experiences into the content of my journey when our three adult children returned to live with us.

It relates to a personal story of an incident that happened in our household. One evening I was looking for something to cook for dinner and found some fish in the freezer. Not giving it much thought, I prepared it for dinner. Little did I realize that this was a *special* fish. This particular fish in question had recently been caught by one of my daughters on a fishing trip, and she was saving it to eat at another time.

Well, all hell broke loose when my daughter realized that the fish I was just about to eat was her *special* fish! She exclaimed, "Who stole my fish?" I felt so guilty that when I owned up, I did not even want to eat the fish anymore, which made the situation even worse as my daughter was visibly upset and responded, "You not only cooked *my* fish, now you're not even going to eat it!"

The consequence of not labeling food items stored in a shared space led to a genuine mistake. However, it demonstrates how a relatively minor incident could make everyone feel uncomfortable and cause tension. My daughter was going through a complete change in her lifestyle at the time. She had been out of the house for nine years already. She had been away from the family and dealing with the accountability of independence that comes with it. Moving back was a big adjustment for her. Fortunately, we were able to look back and laugh about this silly but significant story together.

Within our demographic of friends, many have had their adult children move back home. Similarly, we had all entered this new arrangement blindly, not considering all the implications. Physical spaces and finances were easy for us to deal with, and we worked out the rest along the way. Our experience turned out pretty well, considering some difficulties. Our adult children achieved their goals, and we all managed to keep our sanity. Of course, there were some hiccups along the way, but we dealt with those as they came up, and more importantly, we also had a lot of fun together!

The experience our friends and we had with our adult children, combined with research, was the motivating factor to write this book. Including the realization of the necessity of a book to help guide us back then would have been greatly accepted!

1

NAVIGATING YOUR REACTION

Listening is not merely hearing, it is receiving the message that is being sent to you. Listening is reacting. Listening is being affected by what you hear. Listening is letting it land before you react. Listening is letting your reaction make a difference. Listening is active. –Michael Shurtleff

When approached by your adult child, the reaction you have to their request to ask you if they can move back home is an integral part of this process. If you have developed close relationships with your children, then perhaps this request would not be unexpected, and you would have had time to prepare. This could be beneficial in having had some time to gauge your response. It can be a big surprise when it comes out of the blue. Not every parent/adult-child relationship is close for various reasons. Feelings that may arise from your reaction to hearing about this suggestion of moving back home might jolt you or surprise you. Take this opportunity to accept that you may experience many feelings (both negative and positive) and that these are expected emotions!

Feelings of guilt should be set aside if the advent of your adult children moving back home does not suit you. You might be at the stage of needing this time for your partner and yourself or might not be able to afford the extra mouths to support. Negative feelings are part of the whole process and are allowed to be felt. How will you ever be able to go through life only with positive feelings? It is just not possible. The importance of embracing all your feelings and reaching a decision that is the right one for you cannot be stressed enough. We all are victims of our sense of obligation, and the trick is to determine what these obligations are and still retain a balance with what is good for you.

UNDERSTANDING EXPECTATIONS

Maintaining mutual respect is the first step toward understanding each other's expectations. It is a common habit for many of us to blur the difference between goals and expectations. Expectations are defined as a strong belief that something will happen. This is different from the goals we set, which should be a series of planned, measurable time-framed steps toward something we want to achieve. Emphasis is placed on wanting to understand the adult child's goals and reasons for returning to live with us. Applying this strategy will enable everyone to keep track of progress and adjust these time frames as necessary. Defining and understanding the goals set to be achieved at the beginning of the journey together will help mitigate any conflict in the future.

Having meaningful conversations with each other will help set some goals which will allow you to work together towards achieving them. Goals may need to be negotiated and agreed upon as you will all be living in the same house. For instance, your adult child may have set some long-term goals requiring them to stay for two years, and you feel that this may be too long for them to stay with you. Be clear in stating what you need, as well as why. Being respectful of each other is the key motivating factor. Honesty about your expectations will help you find a clear path to agreement.

Discussions about which goals need to be achieved and how to meet them are essential to the conversations you need to have as a family. Awareness of the reactions that surface and paying heed to each person's needs for every situation during these conversations can help identify what will formulate your desired action plan.

This process cannot be rushed through, and it may take a few meetings to identify everyone's needs. It is also likely that even when you think you have completed your "list," some more items will crop up as you go along. Be open to the game plan changing along the way and remember to be flexible. Again, this highlights the necessity of being open and honest with each other and having a process to follow in dealing with issues that may arise, making the process much smoother.

IDENTIFYING THE PROS AND CONS

Taking time to respond to your adult child's request instead of reacting quickly is a healthy habit to try to stick to. One of the best ways to analyze the impact of any decision reached is to make a list of the pros and cons to give you an idea of the impact of your response. You will probably create this list with your partner or spouse, being mindful that each person may come from an entirely different perspective. It is suggested that your adult child make their list of pros and cons, then sit together and discuss it. You may be surprised at some of the comparative ones, and perhaps some that you had no idea were relevant to yourself and your adult child.

When using these lists as a tool for the work that needs to be done, be mindful of doing it with compassion and caring for one another to reach well-informed and comfortable decisions together.

Here are some examples of the pros that could relate to parents and adult children:

- An opportunity to strengthen relationships with each other during this time

When your children are growing up, they are far more focused on developing their friendships, and now those bonds would more likely have been formed, leaving an opportunity for parent and child to have an unexpected return to forging a new parent–adult-child relationship while living together. Apart from this, there is also emotional support needed from each other from time to time. This is immeasurable in the benefits of having someone close by you can trust who knows the real you. Being able to just be yourself without judgment and with the certainty of love for one another is incomparable.

- Assisting your adult children to become more financially stable

This is the most common reason adult children come home; however, depending on how it is dealt with, this can be both a pro and a con. Focusing on the pro could pave the way for them to get out of crippling debt, save for a home deposit, and have some savings growing in the bank. This will be more easily achieved by paying less rent and reducing overheads for a period of time. This is only attainable by being realistic about your financial situation. You could also be helping them develop a more realistic view of the importance of saving, a valuable life skill.

- More people share living expenses in the household

With much of the research indicating that moving back home is due to financial constraints, sharing household expenses can be instrumental in taking the pressure off everyone. This is circumstantial, and much would depend on the parents' financial stability. Perhaps they do not need any financial contribution. What is constructive when it comes to money is to consider a nominal amount to be paid towards living expenses, even if the parents do not need it. This money can be put aside to boost their savings or something similar. It is beneficial for them to feel responsible and worthy of their contribution to the household. This can also be a period when the adult child has the advantage of improving their credit rating for future loans that may be needed to build a house, etc., without the added pressure of paying high rentals and living expenses.

- Benefiting from sharing endless household tasks

Not only is this a definite pro for everyone, but if everybody pulls their weight equally and does their fair share, it is helpful and leaves everyone with some extra free time. That is rare in this busy world we live in! When your child has become an adult, there are more things that they can help with, which can give a sense of fulfillment in being able to play a positive role in their parent's life. Using their skills to contribute positively to everyone's benefit in the household will give them a great sense of value. This could be anything from their advanced technical skills and culinary abilities to their expertise in the garden!

In our household, preplanning our meals suited us and was an excellent option for increasing participation and lessening the never-ending task of preparing meals in the evening. We made use of the services that provided menu plans and ingredients delivered to the house at the beginning of the week, and we all took turns at meal preparation and cleaning up, which helped to even the balance. Here are some points to ponder:

- Helping them to reassess their career opportunities

Having the right set of circumstances to work for fulfillment rather than just working for that salary at the end of the month needed to pay the bills is a great benefit. Offering this opportunity while they are at home could also allow for additional savings to grow for them while their needs for whatever work they have chosen to do are being achieved. Despite this, it could also potentially be an opportunity for the adult child to pursue an internship that may not have been possible while living away from home and take advantage of this opportunity to either upskill themselves or retrain for a new career direction.

- Perceptions are changing with views on adult children moving back home

There is less judgment, resulting in this return to the parents' home being looked upon more positively. The value placed on solid and supportive family units is instrumentally positive and very fortunate for those with this support structure. Living together could also result in learning good lessons from each other as adults about how goals are set and met. This journey together can enhance their shift to assuming responsibilities as an adult and should not be viewed as a negative factor.

- Moving back to what is known and comfortable has considerable benefits

Depending on the circumstances, this can be a very positive factor experienced for the adult child coming home. Not only will it give some comfort financially, but it will also do so emotionally. There is also a gift of reconnecting with an existing childhood support network from friends to perhaps other members of the family that may still live in the neighborhood. These support networks could be from the regular shop around the corner to the tree they planted in the garden. Feeling secure and safe in an environment can only inspire confidence and motivation for what lies ahead, no matter the challenges.

Processing the Cons

The ease of slipping back into a parent and child relationship is the undeniable challenge everyone will face at some stage. Being consistently aware that the relationship has changed between parent and adult child must be at the forefront of all decisions and behaviors. There is no quick fix for habits, and being a parent is the most challenging job in the world with no manual! Nothing is perfect, but the parent's home is a safety net. To be able to effectively tackle some of the cons that may surface from this arrangement, consider the following:

- Loss of independence for the adult child and coming back to live under another set of rules

The loss of independence can create an upheaval of emotions for your adult child. They may feel they have gone somewhat *backward* by moving back into their childhood home as an adult, and parents will also need to adapt their behaviors. The adult child must ensure they do not detract from the reality that the family home is no longer theirs and that it has now changed to just the parent's home since moving out. It needs to be clear. There may be circumstances where adult children who did not expect change and when they come back home and are faced with changes, may find these differences challenging to accept or even acknowledge.

Habits and expectations they had as a child living in their parent's house may resurface. They may be experiencing anxiety, feeling inadequate, and disappointed in their inability to have achieved a goal. Moving back home may exacerbate these feelings. Even though it is becoming more common and more readily accepted to move back in with your parents, there continues to be a stigma attached to it. Being sensitive to this and talking about it helps by being clear that this process is a plan of action that has been put in place to create a benefit and that it is not a freeloading time; it is a time of action with a clear strategy.

- The importance of redefining boundaries and enabling privacy for both parents and adult children

The realization for the adult child that their childhood home is not the same as it was when they lived there can be a bit of a shock to their system. It will set challenges for both parent and adult child to overcome. It is finding that balance where the adult child feels at home but with the awareness that it is not their home. Parents may struggle with the adaptation of not parenting as they did in the past, such as with setting a reasonable time to come home, etc. The essence of it all is constant communication about what is going on inside your head.

Not only have the parents changed, but so have the adult children, and it will be a time of acknowledgment and acceptance of each other's differences. Being mutually respectful of each other's privacy and space is critical. It cannot be stressed enough to always be ready to listen to each other. Grab this opportunity you have been given to make the most of all the quality time you will have together.

- Acknowledging the return to the home may be due to a hindrance and not a choice

More often than not, it is the last choice reached by your adult child to move back home. The lack of self-esteem is probably the most significantly affected emotion that can be taxing on those around you. Being honest and open with the problems that created this move back and the plan that has been put in place to improve the situation. All of this is predominantly and ultimately designed to lead them back to their independence and is a part of a caring and nurturing process. It is not all about hard and fast rules and pressure. Allowing each other the space to deal with the invasion of your space takes patience. Everyone should be mindful of the importance of self-care and taking *time out* to *just be*. Activities such as meditation, yoga, gardening, or reading a book—whatever settles your mind to put you back into a positive thinking mode. Nobody can tackle problems when they are in a negative state of mind.

- Financial Consequences

Up to now, parents would have had ultimate freedom of how to spend their money, as would the adult children. When they move back home, this changes as both parties can view how the other is spending their money, which can cause tension. For example, in your view, if an adult child living at home suddenly purchases a top-of-the-range costly and perhaps unnecessary item but says they cannot afford to contribute to household expenses, this is a dangerous place to be. Resentment will rise and create an untenable situation for all.

It is vital to have the financial contributions clear from the start. No matter what the end decision is on how to use this income, be it towards actual expenses or placed into a savings account (unbeknown to them) to be utilized later. For the most part, the main reason for coming back home is some financial instability, so this is an opportunity to address this issue and find a clear path toward a successful outcome.

Even though you want to help, beware of making your adult child dependent on you. You may be saving for retirement or paying off your mortgage and will not want to go backward. Stay the course with your financial plan and security and take care not to put this at risk. If circumstances lead to you having to help support your adult child, it will be harder for you and your partner or spouse, especially if they are not contributing much financially. There is a vast difference between helping and enabling your adult child.

If you do not have clear guidelines, it could cause all sorts of issues that, if they are left unaddressed, could brew a strong undercurrent and blow up at an inopportune moment.

Establishing these reasonable timelines for what is needed and when their portion of a contribution to household expenses is due must be clarified. Perhaps this could be the first month or two for free, and then it kicks in with the agreed timelines being activated and what their contributions and expectations are. It has to work for you as this is your household. It could be a flat rate, or they perhaps could buy certain items. The critical element to consider here is to provide your adult children with the tools they need to be financially independent and secure without your financial help.

Our adult children contributed a weekly amount towards food, power, and utilities; however, it was at a reduced rate to what the market was charging. We also considered their circumstances as one had a part-time job but was searching for full-time employment and so contributed less at that time.

- Storage warfare

Perhaps you may have scaled down or just do not have the room for all their stuff. Reaching an agreement on how the possessions they move in with will impact your home is essential. No one wants to feel crowded or experience tripping over stuff that ends up *in the way*. Not sorting this out could create unnecessary stress if not dealt with right from the start.

My husband and I lived in a three-bedroomed townhouse when our adult children asked us to come home. Fortunately, we did have space available in terms of bedrooms; however, our adult children had to arrange and pay for additional external storage as we simply did not have enough room for all their possessions. Communication and mutual respect continued to be the key to minimizing conflict and maximizing opportunities.

2

HAVING THE TALK

We haven't got a plan so nothing can go wrong. –Spike Milligan

The quote is quite ironic as I am a note planner, and plans are needed to create some structure. However, it aims to bring some humor into a somewhat serious topic!

Generally speaking, most parents know when the time comes for their child to want to move back home. This is probably the most critical time when you have that first talk or initial request about it, particularly for those who did not know what they would be presenting to you. Emphasis must be placed on the reasons your child made this decision. Apart from this, be aware of what your concerns are and how it is going to work.

It is essential to have this talk beforehand, or at the very least in the early days of them moving in. A frank and open discussion about what is not acceptable is essential for everyone to be on the same page; for example, no smoking in the house or no loud music late at night. Some of your reasons may seem trivial to your adult children and even others who hear about them, but what is important to remember is to be clear about what you cannot deal with or accept. This is your home, after all, and being clear about what the guidelines you and your partner or spouse require must be communicated right from the start for everyone's sanity. Things may have changed in your home since they left, and they must be aware of this. It is a big step for most adult children to move back home and creating a sense of support and love is vital for everyone to benefit.

There are also some big questions to ask yourself too.

Is your help in any way going to impact your child's growth negatively? The goal for all parents is to prepare them adequately to be able to stand on their own feet and be independent.

Asking these pertinent questions may help to put the situation into perspective on how to move forward.

- What has created this situation for them?
- Is it something beyond their control or have they been irresponsible?
- Will your retirement savings and the like affect your financial status?

Most importantly, it is necessary to be clear that you are offering help and not hindering your child's development. Be open about how helping them affects you without any emotional blackmail, so they have an insight into the reality of your world. Some children have no idea if their parents are struggling to survive. With this new change of circumstances of them moving in, you might have to delay your retirement, dip into your nest egg of savings, and give up a pending trip you had planned; not to mention the effects of having no privacy in your home for you and your spouse anymore. There are so many reasons, and it is advised that you make a list of them that relate to your situation. The reality is that this *boomerang* phenomenon is a growing trend, particularly in the last 10 years and even more so recently. It is a temporary arrangement to assist your adult children in becoming more financially stable and can range from a few months to a few years.

Our adult children had clear goals to achieve before moving back home. One wanted to focus on the intention to save money until the completion of a degree and for a deposit for a house. The other returned from overseas due to the impact of COVID-19 on an industry which was negatively affected, resulting in the need to find new employment.

I am sure that there were mixed emotions for everyone in the household. One of our adult children was processing several different emotions due to a sudden change in career and the abrupt loss of independence. Adjusting takes time. There is no magic formula; the best you can offer is support and patience. It is hard not to get back into the adult-child relationship mode and start caretaking. This may cause a backlash at the time that may appear to be hurtful when they do not accept your care. Remember, they are adjusting to new circumstances and a new adult-adult relationship as well.

WHAT TO EXPECT

As parents of adult children, having a good understanding of your child's expectations for their need for independence will significantly benefit the situation of acknowledging what it was that changed their situation. Knowing what support they need now to deal with this change in their lifestyle of deciding to come home is important. They will more than likely be disappointed in themselves that they were not able to make a success of their venture into the big world, and the last thing they need is harsh judgment. Many who have been out of home for some time might have expected a completely different outcome from what adulthood was meant to be for them. Losing their newfound independence is a challenge they will need to address.

Asking the pertinent question of why they need to come home is reasonable, and they should be able to answer. The primary motivation for this decision should be clear. They should be able to discuss their feelings about what led to this decision and why coming home was the only option for them to consider. From the adult child's perspective, the same applies regarding the parent's expectations and accepting how different it will be living back at home than it was when they were a child.

Feelings may surface that you might not have expected and may take you completely by surprise. Many of us respond too quickly without realizing we have not even listened to the other person's full story yet. Being patient and aware of your feelings, whether anger, fear, frustration, guilt, or anxiety, to mention a few, and to be fully present in how they make you feel is necessary. Be brutally honest and open about your feelings, and also be aware that you can take your time with your response. If you need time to think about it, do so. Always communicate that you cannot verbally express what you are feeling right now and need some time to assimilate your response. There may be a situation where perhaps you were thinking of scaling down and selling the house but had not discussed it yet with your children, and moving back in would potentially change those plans for you. There are always many things to consider. The important point here is to be honest, and if you do not have the answer right away, say so.

RESPOND, DON'T REACT

There is a saying that goes somewhere along the lines of, you are only in control of your reactions, not the situation. This is good advice, particularly when you are hesitant about your child's move back home, which is okay.

As mentioned above, many of us feel compelled to know the answer immediately, but we do not need to. What we do have to do is say that we need time to gather our thoughts. Several discussions are often required to work out a plan. Attaining a balance is what you want to achieve. Even though there will be challenges along the way, there will be great rewards too. Reacting too quickly without thought can sometimes change a situation into a negative one without knowing what it could have been without a harsh reaction. Breathe, think and take the time you need. Remember the importance of listening without interjecting, and resist the urge to correct your adult child while they are speaking to you. Try not to interrupt; it is the most annoying and rude thing. Whatever the outcome, the aim is to be fair to everyone and that all involved feel valued.

KEY STRATEGIES TO IMPLEMENT

Several good strategies can help you navigate through this time of what could be a very emotional one. Most of these listed below will apply to many families, but of course, you will know deep down what will work in your family situation. Adapting these strategies to suit your household is a starting point.

Keeping Your Cool

No matter why your adult child needs to return home for a period, and even if this situation creates some tension or even anger, the most important reaction is to keep your cool. There may be disappointment from both sides of the fence, but it is more likely that your adult child will feel it a bit more. Moving from an independent situation to moving back home is a huge adjustment. Perhaps even asking to move back home is a massive step backward for them, and they may be apprehensive of your reaction.

In today's society, it is becoming much more common for adult children to return home for a period of time. It was not so long ago and still exists in some households today that it was viewed negatively when your adult child moved back home. It was considered a failure, or they were lazy or inadequate. The financial pressures in today's society are becoming so demanding that it is taking longer for young adults to be financially independent. There is also a trend of a growing number of adult children who may delay moving out and only leave in their late 20s and 30s. Focusing on the tools they need to achieve independence and nurturing them to find the way instead of blowing up at their perceived failures is the way to go.

Setting the Timeline Period

This is not only for the parent's benefit but for the adult child too. It is vital to have some goalposts for how long they expect to live at home, even if these timelines are adjusted. When a timeline has not been set, it will leave both parties in a state of limbo, which is unhealthy for anyone. Being transparent with each other and when the deadline is looming with no change to their situation and letting weeks slide to months and even years without an agreement with each other is unhealthy. It is important to discuss it. When nearing the deadline date and if new timelines need to be set, make ample time to discuss what everyone's needs are and how a new timeline can be agreed upon that is acceptable to everyone.

Creating Boundaries Together

Each household differs in how they raise their children and their boundaries. New boundaries need to be created when your adult child is living back home. Things may have changed in the household since they left, and these need to be communicated as to what is or is not acceptable. Adult children need to understand that their parents have developed a different way of living without them; for many, this might be the first time they have had this opportunity. The whole deal about creating boundaries is to do it together and discuss finding the medium ground where everyone involved feels comfortable with and aware of these boundaries. Some families use business practice strategies to help them with this process. Finding out what works for you and your family is a collaborative and personal journey. Some families will go the route of having a lease or an agreement drawn so everyone is on the same page. This can include all sorts of things, from visitors, unacceptable behavior, responsibilities around the home, the time frame of expected stay, and financial contributions.

Sometimes, adult children are baffled by their parents changing house rules, particularly ones they were used to. This is your choice to do this, not because you are being difficult about it, but because they need to understand these boundaries have been set for a specific reason that is important to you now.

Maintaining Respect for Each Other

Whatever you come up with as a plan for this new phase together, maintaining respect for each other all the time must be one of the most important values in a family. It is well known that respect is earned, and it is a two-way street. Realize that your child is an adult who will want to make their own decisions even though they are living under your roof and that both sides may need to make some adjustments. For example, to come down hard on some rules for your adult child will only lead to resentment. It should instead come by way of respect for each other, instilling a system of checking in on each other to advise expected time home, and so on. Bristling with fury over a cooked meal going cold, but not having communicated that you were making dinner for the family at a particular time, is unreasonable. The same goes for respect for areas of your home to allow for privacy of respectfulness of each other's space. Do not expect to be involved in every moment of your child's day. Making compromises is part of it, but not to the detriment of your values and important things that matter to you.

Managing the Disappointments

You may be fortunate to sail through all this with no disappointments or even moments of blazing anger, but it is unusual for everyone to get along all the time. It boils down to good communication and setting boundaries to help manage disappointments. If, for example, you have loaned them some money to establish something and it does not work out, it is not beneficial to anyone to be angry about it if you did not set clear parameters at the beginning of the process. If you wanted to be involved from the beginning in seeing how it was evolving, then this needs to be clarified ahead of time to prevent any strife. In other words, do not micromanage or place unreasonable terms upon loans offered. Decide to either do it or not to avoid getting disappointed.

Having Regular Family Meetings

This might seem a bit over the top, but it does have some great benefits. It is not only for keeping the parameters clear and having a platform to sort out any issues before they become complex and challenging to deal with but also to keep strengthening the family unit. Keeping these meetings short and calm, even applying an agenda to them, can help keep things on track, so everyone has an opportunity to voice their concerns. It is about ensuring the conversations are on point while not being too dogmatic either—this is not a formal board meeting. Allowing conversations to flow without going off point is integral. This is also not a time for the parent to do all the talking either! These gatherings work better with screen-free time so that there are no distractions. If anything has not been resolved, make notes to address at the next meeting and ensure everyone knows when that is and the importance of attending. Adding a regular family activity at the end of the meeting, such as a board game afterward, is an excellent way to smooth the waters and have fun.

Contributing to the Household Expenses

Your financial circumstances will determine how much monetary support you can offer your child. The subject of money often brings out the worst in people, so again, clarity of what is expected must be communicated. If your child is not working and has no income, they should contribute to the household in other ways. It is all about accountability, responsibility, and, most of all, self-worth. Some families take the rent their children are paying and save it for them (unbeknown to them) to give them later, perhaps as a deposit for a house or towards a significant outlay. Some families put it into their retirement fund. Others work out an amount according to their earnings or even split it between a household contribution and savings. There are no right or wrong answers. These are merely suggestions; it will depend on your family and your situation to determine the most suitable one.

Our adult children contributed financially to household expenses. There is mutual benefit to be gained here. Not only does it contribute to achieving self-worth for the adult child, but it will also provide some financial stability for the parents.

3

COMMUNICATION IS THE KEY

Don't wait until everything is just right. It will never be perfect. There will always be challenges, obstacles, and less-than-perfect conditions. So what. Get started now. With each step you take, you will grow stronger and stronger, more and more skilled, more and more self-confident, and more and more successful. –Mark Victor Hansen

This quote puts communication into perspective for me as it is a skill that just becomes better and easier the more you practice it with each other. Not speaking and listening to each other will only antagonize the situation, as nobody will know what is expected from them if they have not been told.

After processing the pros and cons, we agreed to the new live-in arrangement for a defined period with the objective in mind to enable our adult children to achieve specific goals.

We were blessed that our adult children continued to live by and own the same values they had learned from us growing up. Therefore, we didn't have any real value-related issues that had to be negotiated. On occasions, both parties would gently remind each other about certain habits that were beginning to get on each other's nerves. But by and large, this was communicated without arguments, tension, or conflict. We did not schedule family meetings because we all ate at the table for the evening meal on most occasions and took this opportunity to air any grievances and just have a regular catch-up with each other.

SOME IDEAS TO CONSIDER TO HELP WITH COMMUNICATION

Something to consider is to create a group chat on social media such as Facebook Messenger, WhatsApp, etc., as they are convenient tools to use for communication. This is because everyone gets the same message at the same time; for instance, if someone is going to be home late or not home for dinner. Our world has become one where it has become the norm to want an instant result, and keeping up with (and making use of) technology has its benefits, although it will never replace the real deal of being face to face!

When the day approaches for when your adult child is due to move in, and depending on how you operate as a parent, you may be one of those that have spent hours getting everything ready for them. The opposite could happen, with you waiting for them to arrive and clear out *their room* of the stuff you had piled in there as it may have become a study, sewing room, or just a spare room. Neither of these is better than the other; it is personal. Some adult children take it personally that *their room* has been changed to something else.

This is all part of the journey of accepting the inevitable changes that will be experienced, which should be communicated with each other as to how it will all work. An idea of how this new living arrangement is envisaged by everyone involved should be discussed.

After identifying your feelings and being practical about the pros and cons of having your adult child live back home, now is the time to communicate all these concerns with them. If you keep it all inside and do not speak about your problems, no one will understand your needs. Commit to your decisions or adaptations to have them back in your home and stick to them. Bemoaning that your adult child is now in your sewing room, for instance, will achieve very little in making them feel welcome. At the same time, your adult child should be made aware of your willingness to sacrifice a special place for them. The behavior of acknowledging it and appreciating it is to be welcomed.

Sometimes, talking through the concerns with your adult child or partner will achieve a result without much effort. This does not happen all the time though! Learning the ability to communicate clearly with each other is an ongoing process. Communication is like a circle; it never ends. For some, it is easier to write things down to refer to and then move forward, which may help keep you on track with your needs.

WHAT SHOULD NON-NEGOTIABLES BE?

Being crystal clear about what is not acceptable will help toward creating a harmonious home environment. The trick is consistency. If you allow something some of the time and then freak out when it happens at another time, it is unfair to everyone involved. Respect should be right at the top of the list, not only for this new phase but as an instilled value.

This is where a pre-move-in plan is created and where you begin to set prospective boundaries is helpful as a starting point. Being considerate of each other's needs and space is paramount. This may sound a bit dogmatic, but having it written down and outlining the requirements makes it easier to refer back to when and if problems arise. Even if you have not tackled this step before your adult child moves in, it is never too late to do it.

This is the time to define those boundaries for each other. Yours may include loud music parameters, staying up till the wee hours, foul language, drugs, alcohol, etc. Discuss the mutual expectations you have of each other and what the house rules are. They may have changed in the home from what they once were to what your adult child thinks they may still be. Communicate this clearly, as this living situation is a new one. They are not returning as children. They are coming into your home as an adult, and this comes with specific responsibilities.

There may be some resentment from your adult child being told to stick to the boundaries you want to enforce. There may even be a feeling of resentment, as they are an adult now and perhaps feel they do not need to be told what to do anymore and make their own decisions. The logic here is simple: This is your home, that you have opened up to them to help them out.

Suppose you have taken the time to consider most of the variables. In that case, this will help reduce any possible misunderstandings and the potential of creating friction between everyone who lives in the house. Consider what is courteous and considerate for each other, rather than it being a set of rules and regulations.

Clarify the rental amount and when it is to be paid and be reasonable. Have an idea of how long they intend on staying and their long-term and short-term goals so you are best prepared to know how you can assist. This whole process of the initial discussion is to create a mental plan of what you envisage the situation to be like. It is preferable to document this to minimize confusion and have something to refer back to. A template is included at the end of this book.

Most, if not all of us, feel a lot more secure in a new venture whatever that may be, when we have clarity of what it entails and more importantly, what is not negotiable. It is often a more straightforward process, to begin with the non-negotiables and clear those up first.

If your adult child is not working and stays up late into the early hours, disturbing the peace for the rest of the household, this is disrespectful, particularly if you are still working, and will, in the end, cause upset. Sometimes it is frustrating when what we think is a common courtesy is not regarded the same way by others' eyes —particularly when it comes to our offspring!

These non-negotiables are very important to help create balance in your home, even with the obligations you may feel to provide your adult child with a roof over their head. Leaving it be and not dealing with these issues will fester and create massive disruption. Being direct without making excuses or reasoning why you feel a particular *rule* is important is vital.

Going blind with no prior discussions or agreement with each other is quite different from "going with the flow." The flow would still require some sort of direction.

CONTINUING THE CONVERSATION

Understanding that this return to home is an ideal time to help your adult child develop improved skills for adapting to adult life with your guidance. The key word is guidance, as this is all you can do. As adults, they will expect adult privileges which is perfectly acceptable. It must be reiterated that their choices should not undermine anyone else in the household when taken.

Having a plan of action is essential so goals can be set, and then you can strategize how to achieve them. This is not only about money, although it does play a big part. Your adult child must understand your situation, which would have very different outcomes depending on whether you are still working or retired. Beware of dipping into retirement savings as this could have drastic and detrimental effects on your future.

The following three scenarios have different consequences for the parent. In the first instance, you may be in a secure financial position and able to give them money. Secondly, you could consider an option of it being a loan to them, which could either have interest added to it or not. Thirdly, perhaps you could save the money they contribute to the household, either for you to use or maybe to gift back to them later. All of these options will create different outcomes. What will work for one family may not work for another.

Considering your needs will be crucial in moving forward regarding the financial conversation. Feelings of guilt sometimes can be an overwhelming emotion for a parent, as we all just want the best for our children. Guilt can lead to resentment because when responsibility knocks on the door, and we succumb to it, resentment will follow right behind it! Giving in and agreeing to something against your values, principles, and something you both have decided on is quite simply not being responsible for yourself. Be aware and cautious of being pulled down the "made to feel guilty" path.

The Pre-move-in Plan

Drawing up your pre-move-in plan where prospective boundaries are considered can include the following and vary from household to household. This is just to give you a bit of direction to create your own. It is a discussion document that may change quite a bit until you reach a final one that you have negotiated and agreed upon. Think of it as part of a negotiation process.

Perhaps start the document with a brief outline of how you envisage this situation and how it is seen ideally in your eyes.

1. Mutual expectations and house rules must be clear from the beginning.

Being courteous with each other is fundamental when instilling house rules. This could range from agreeing to calling if they will be late or not coming home that evening, so no one worries unnecessarily about the other, to not parking in your spot! Have a structure for responsibilities like jotting down toilet paper on the shopping list stuck on the fridge when they see you are on the last roll, taking out the trash, feeding the animals, or creating meal plans. It will and must fit in with what makes you comfortable. Perhaps in the past, the mom always cooked dinner, which is now a shared role with everyone in the household. Expectations can be tricky and need to be spoken about a lot!

2. List your primary concerns, why you have them, and why they are important.

Many parents struggle with the fear of enabling their adult children and preventing them from standing on their own two feet by offering too much help. Adult children are adults, not children; they must assume responsibility for themselves. Striking a balance between you and them and what works in your family unit with what assistance you can offer is the prize you are seeking. We all tend to fall into the bad habit of comparisons at times but try not to go down that road, as it can harm relationships. Focus on what your family values are and what is important. Work together to establish what you both need from each other without taking advantage of the situation. Always be open about the challenges faced and if you are feeling hurt or taken advantage of.

3. Counter these concerns with suggestions to improve and restructure what is troubling.

Using the example from the previous point, ask your children to participate and share their thoughts on this concern of yours. It is frustrating to hear someone constantly complain about something but never offer a suggested alternative. Even if you do not know what could work to change the situation, discuss it, and through talking about it, you will be surprised at how solutions will surface.

4. There should be shared and private spaces for everyone in the household

When parents reach that stage of no children in the house, the norm often changes, and sometimes this is a bit of a surprise for adult children. Being clear about the value of privacy, the respect for each other's boundaries, and what areas of the home are common or shared. An adult child may think it is ridiculous that dad wants the blinds drawn at a particular time of day without even considering why. It could be that he does not want the harsh sun on his wine collection, which is a valid reason. What does matter is that the adult child must not be a child about it, and the parent must be clear about their explanations. Respect for their parents' home is paramount. It works both ways too. Respect your adult child's privacy and accept that you will not be involved in everything they do, even if they live in your house.

5. What to do if it is not working and the situation is becoming unbearable

This has to be included. So, if it is not working out, you would have already discussed how to figure out a process for them to move out so that it does not end up in quarrels and hurtful behavior. Family is important, and retaining bonds with each other is the ultimate goal. Even if you cannot live with each other, you can still love each other. Some questions can be asked that may help remedy a breakdown in the situation at home, such as:

- Are the boundaries created not clear enough?
- Are the expectations unreasonable?
- Have the money issues not been clarified?

Gritting your teeth and waiting for the day they move out can damage your relationship. Instead, be open about the issues, and find ways to resolve problems peacefully to maintain your family relationships.

6. Non-negotiables are very important to clarify.

This has already been covered in some depth earlier in the chapter but is on the list again as a reminder not to leave it out of your plan.

7. Responsibilities in the household are for everyone to share.

There are not many that love housework! Setting up a roster can help keep everyone on track with their duties. Again, you need to be upfront with the expectations of what is required. More people in the house make more mess, so more must be done to keep the house functioning smoothly. It is also beneficial to this roster to give each person at least one day where they do nothing! The benefits of sharing the load must be taken advantage of.

8. Goals and how to set them and how to achieve them.

Helping your child revisit their perceived goals is probably the most valuable life lesson you can share with them. Learning how to do this effectively without offending is the trick! Timing is crucial, and it is never a good idea to bombard them with questions about how things are going when they are stressed, rushed, or just about to head out the door. Explain that goals are a target to be achieved. However, goals may need to be adjusted due to life's changing circumstances to keep them realistic.

9. Setting time limits and the exit strategy that everyone agrees to.

Every situation will have different parameters on what these time limits are until they move out. For example, the goal could be:

- when a defined amount of savings is reached
- a specified number of months in gainful employment
- a set period of weeks or months (even years in some cases).

What is important here is that there is a distinct motivating factor to reach the goal of moving out and into their own home. Being flexible and allowing time limits to be adjusted is perfectly okay. Just be clear about what these adjustments mean to everyone involved and what process will be followed when adjustments are made.

Some things come across our paths that are unexpected, like the COVID-19 pandemic that threw many of our lives into turmoil, and we all had to adapt to drastic changes.

In closing, about drawing up your pre-move-in plan, try not to be too rigid in your demands without compromising. Compromise is not giving in. It is finding a proper balance. This document or agreement might seem unnecessary or tedious to some families, but what is to be stressed about these agreements is that they are living documents and can be adapted as changes happen. The emphasis is to keep communication channels open, honest, respectful, and loving.

4

SETTING COMMON GROUND

How far you go in life depends on your being tender with the young, compassionate with the aged, sympathetic with the striving, and tolerant of the weak and strong. Because someday in your life you will have been all of these. –George Washington Carver

Finding common ground will be much simpler for everyone if the non-negotiables, boundaries, and expectations of each other have been clearly laid out. The most common stumbling block is adjusting our behavior patterns with each other. As challenging as it may be for the parent to hold back on parenting the adult child, the same applies to the adult child to behave as an adult now and not a child.

The boundaries and non-negotiables that were previously agreed upon might have to be reconsidered. Maintaining an equilibrium that is fair and acceptable to everyone is what you are aiming for. Being reasonable and honest about why some of them will be non-negotiable, and presenting why they are, may be necessary.

Living together again requires a lot of giving and taking from each other. At times in my household, I felt we almost created what can be described as a type of dance flow in the house. The kitchen and the lounge are the best examples of this dance-flow experience. Someone would be in the kitchen eating breakfast and preparing their lunch for work, and just as they head out, someone else would move into that space and continue to do what they had to do (taking their place on the dance floor so to speak!)

Everyone in the same space can sometimes create challenging moments of being on top of one another and crowding each other, which can become quite frustrating. Finding your flow to your household that works for everyone, and creating your family *dance*, will help to keep the peace.

YOUR ADULT CHILD MAY HAVE CONCERNS

Allowing time to be able to express concerns without fear of judgment or reprisal will afford you both great leaps ahead in the process. Sometimes we are so focused on what we want or need that it may cloud our perception of how this could affect someone else.

Being compassionate and understanding each other's needs are indispensable in moving forward with agreements that are acceptable to everyone involved. This may also be having to compromise with each other, which may be challenging. It is not a case of being the one who has to give in or let another person walk all over them and being allowed to manipulate decisions. This is nowhere near a compromise. Navigating these feelings gently and honestly will help to avoid conflict, particularly when both sides feel strongly about their point of view.

Whatever the concerns your adult child raises, these must be reasonable and not just because they thought it would be different, and now it must be. Accepting a change to something that has always been a particular way, or a way you expected it to be, and now it is not, is sometimes difficult to accept. It could be a simple thing to something very complex. Remember that the little things can fester if left, leading to more significant problems. Typically, annoying habits for either party may include wet washing left in the machine, dirty dishes in the sink, personal items scattered all over the house, or lack of privacy. It is not an opening to nitpick at issues but rather to sort out more minor problems as they arise with openness and by remaining tactful at all times. The aim is to prevent these things that annoy us from growing into massive issues that are difficult to deal with.

It is pertinent that your adult child realizes that the way they behaved as a child in the home when they were growing up is just not going to cut it when being an adult in the same house. Growing up is their responsibility, and the values that were instilled in them as children by their parents should help them become responsible adults.

Building on Conversations About Concerns Raised

"The only way forward is through" is a saying many of us have heard. It is quite surprising that an effective outcome is often reached when the work is done together in a positive way to find a resolution. Keeping these channels of communication fluid with each other could even result in a different outcome than either of you expected. It could also result in even creating some additional boundaries or discovering unknown common ground that may need to be reached, which in the end, suits everyone even better. Approaching things with a positive attitude can lead to marvelous results if you let it!

Being negative or critical can be hard to avoid, particularly if you feel cornered, unheard, or frustrated. The best thing to do when things start to go pear-shaped with a conversation is to take a break and return with an open mind and calm attitude. Do whatever works for you, such as a walk, a bike ride, meditation, or a nice bubble bath. You know what works to settle your mind. Picking up fresh where you left off in a negative situation can turn the tide effectively more often than not. The emphasis here is to return to dealing with the issue at hand. Being kind to one another, particularly after some harsh words, is a step in the right direction to begin the conversation again and find a way to resolve an issue.

Standing Your Ground

No matter how you run your household and define what is acceptable and what is not, once you have figured this out, stand your ground. If something needs to be changed, talk about it. Allow time for adaptation, but not an endless time limit either!

Whatever the reasons you have established for being non-negotiable about something, stick to them if they are reasonable and important to you. Being open to constructive criticism and being willing to re-evaluate decisions is not giving in—it is, again, being reasonable. If there is resistance, asking for alternatives to your non-negotiables is another solution to find a way through. Just saying no to something is not enough; it needs to have substance as to why it is a no. When your children become adults, they will likely question your motives even more than they did as teenagers. It is a huge shift when children become adults, and sometimes they might even slip into the role of parenting the parents! This can also lead to some serious conflict as parents are used to being the ones in charge.

Taking a big step back and listening to their opinions does help soothe a pending argument. In turn, they should return due respect by listening to your views. Be clear that your values in your home have not changed; as they will be living here, they will need to adapt to them if they have changed. Also, do not be too rigid in what you want or think is right. Sometimes, your adult children surprise you and open your eyes to a specific of yours that might need a change!

Avoiding conflict is what everyone wants, more often than not. Those looking for conflict are exceptionally difficult people to deal with, which is another book. For this book, the focus is on avoiding conflict and finding a structure that works for everyone.

Identifying conflict is the first step toward rectifying the situation. We all have different personalities, and life would be pretty boring if we agreed on everything. Someone challenging you is not necessarily wrong, but if you do not handle the conflict well, it could turn about-face rather quickly and become unpleasant for everyone. Acceptance of lessons to be learned from conflicts can be rewarding. Admitting when you have been wrong and apologizing is sometimes difficult, particularly if you are a little stubborn, but taking the time to reflect on what made an issue an issue is needed.

There are varying types of conflicts, but all relate to differences of opinion, even if the ultimate goal may be the same. The pitfall of conflicts is the doorway that can open to behavior that borders on bullying or even teasing. This can be exceptionally hurtful to the receiver. Joking continuously and being sarcastic about someone else is not fair if it is something that has become a bit of a habit. Being caring and gentle about each other's feelings shows respect, but you still need to have a voice and communicate your concerns. Conflicts can often arise from being ignored or ridiculed about something you feel is relevant to you.

Family members usually will have the same or similar values, but not always. Sometimes if there are differences in these values, it can create a powerful conflict that can be very hard to diffuse. It most often will end up agreeing to disagree while moving forward amicably. If this situation arises in your household, it will be up to you to determine the outcome as your house and your rules apply to something you feel very strongly about. How issues are dealt with, from the kitchen being left in a mess and people not cleaning up after themselves to how visitors are treated in the home, can also lead to conflicts. Tackling how to deal with these differences will often relate to values again. Keeping egos in check, not allowing them to dominate or personally attack each other with harsh words, is ideally what you want to prevent. Keeping your communication transparent with no hidden agenda will give you the most effective result that can resolve an issue and present a window of opportunity to understand each other's differences. Also, find a way to accept them without diminishing your principles.

Sometimes, you may need to draw back from conflict, which is not bad, as long as it is for self-preservation where you need time to calm your mind and perhaps let tempers settle before attempting to tackle the issue. Other times, the argument is meaningless in the bigger sphere of things and not worth the effort of getting upset. The main concern about withdrawing from a conflict is ensuring you are doing it for the right reasons. If it is regularly done for any issue that surfaces, it can feel like you are in a constant war zone and will be exhausting for everyone. Avoidance of important matters by just brushing them under the carpet will eventually create more significant problems in the long term. In the same instance, if you are too passive and keep agreeing or going along with something you are not entirely happy with, it will eventually also have adverse effects.

The same goes for being too aggressive with your ideals. Even if you are 100% correct, forcing your opinion onto your adult child when they think they are right will result in a serious bumping of heads! Keeping the conversation respectful and polite will go a long way, particularly if you are faced with rudeness and disrespect. The best way to deal with this situation is to rise above it and not retaliate in anger. Being willing to collaborate to dive into problem-solving together to reach a compromise in a difficult situation has an immeasurable reward for developing a well-balanced parent and adult-child relationship.

When it comes to conflicts and trying to solve them, we often employ strategies such as the blame game or not acknowledging the issue raised and counter-attacking with a defensive response. This will only result in going around in circles with no positive outcome. Keep your problems specific and deal with them as they arise; otherwise, you may end up with no resolutions and have the same arguments repeatedly.

Ultimately, everyone wants to live in a happy home environment, and no one should lose sight of this. Having disagreements is healthy in a balanced life, but it is essential to consider how you deal with these and move forward together.

Going for a walk was one of the best distractions when I felt uncomfortable or frustrated with a situation. The more frustrated I was, the longer the walk was! It always worked for me; by the time I returned, I had a different perspective and saw things in a new light. One night in particular, after processing during a walk, I approached my home and saw the cars that belonged to my adult children in my driveway. This was a powerful realization that I was fortunate to have my adult children home; they were safe and well. God reminded me how blessed I was, and I felt an overwhelming sense of peace and joy that they were there.

5

WELCOME HOME!—YOUR CHILD MOVES BACK IN

In family life, love is the oil that eases friction. –Eva Burrows

The time has come for your adult child, or perhaps even their children, to move back in. It is likely to be a highly emotionally charged time, and you need to be in tune with your feelings. Following through with the suggestions given in the earlier chapters of the book should offer some reprieve if situations get out of control. Maintaining respect and love for each other should always be at the forefront.

It may take a few days to get into the swing of things with your new relationship with each other. Keep those communication channels open and honest from day one, instead of an attitude of *leaving it till later* or perhaps *saying nothing to keep the peace.* These behaviors should be obliterated from this new living relationship together.

This is also a precious time of new beginnings, with all of you being given a unique opportunity to enjoy exploring the fantastic newness of an adult-adult relationship under the same roof. There will be many moments of extraordinary times together; hopefully, these will outweigh any difficult ones!

Becoming a parent is one of the most important roles we will ever fill, but it is also the toughest! Our children have known us all their lives and know exactly what buttons to push to get reactions. Be mindful of these behavior patterns that result in conflict that can become destructive and create an imbalance in your household.

Not only is this a second chance for them, but also another opportunity for you to encourage some productive habits into their lifestyle. Society has not helped in the creation of an instant gratification attitude. Our daily lives are so fast, and the internet has created the urgency of obtaining information needed immediately. It is almost as if patience has sometimes gone out of the window! Some people have referred to this generation (those born after 2010) as the *snowflake generation* (Cambridge Dictionary, 2022), meaning they are too easily offended. This is quite derogatory but does have a bit of truth to it too. Generational changes will always raise some issues forever in the future, and the crux of the matter is that only that generation at the time they are in it will know what it feels like to be in it. Other generations will only have an idea and an opinion of what they think it is like. It is quite a complex issue but something to be mindful of.

IDENTIFYING PERSONAL SPACE AND BOUNDARIES

Although you have discussed and negotiated this in principle, it is always different when it comes to the real thing! Needs change for everyone due to all sorts of circumstances and being present in the situations and sensitive to each other's needs is integral.

If your personal space has been repeatedly compromised, then it needs to be dealt with. The same goes for the parent crowding their adult child's personal space. Just because it is your house does not mean it is okay to barge into their room without being respectful. A knock on their door if it is closed, and waiting for an answer to come in, is just good manners and respect. This, of course, applies vice versa to everyone else in the household. If boundaries and personal space are undermined, it can bring up many feelings of resentment and anger toward each other. All of this can be easily avoided if you are conscious about being upfront about your personal space and the necessary boundaries to ensure no one is feeling jeopardized.

Never mind all the stuff that comes with them. Deciding on how this will be handled and stored is essential and will depend on how much furniture, boxes, etc., is to be dealt with. Some parents still struggle to deal with keeping their adult children's stuff for years after they have moved out. It is about them taking responsibility for their possessions and finding the best solution. There are many options to consider, from hired storage to perhaps even selling their possessions, saving the money earned, and buying new things when they move out. Much will depend on personal circumstances and space.

In our household, some big questions came up:

- How do we share communal spaces equitably?
- What arrangements can we make to prepare for this?
- Is a pre-agreed schedule the way to go?

Depending on your home layout, and if you have two lounges already existing or have the space to create two lounges, this can make life much easier, especially if small children are involved. It is then clearly defined that one area is theirs and the other is yours. This helps solve so many issues.

On one occasion, we even converted our garage into a living area. It just took popping in a secondhand couch, a couple of bean bags, a small table, a lamp stand, and a rug. There you have it!

Their lounge was an easy process to create and gave them their own cozy space. If things like television, computers, gaming consoles, and music set-ups are required, this can be provided by themselves and add to the reality that this is their own space.

Regarding storage, we had some space available in our house; although we did have to re-organize, it did not impact us negatively by allowing our adult children to store their possessions here. If this is not possible in your home for whatever reason, there are plenty of other options for storage to consider, such as:

- renting storage facilities nearby
- considering rent-a-room where available

These are some packaging ideas that worked for us and ended up reducing the area needed for the storage of bulky items:

- Pack items into clear plastic bins for storage that are clearly labeled so you can see what is in them without having to unpack and repack!
- A great tip is to choose bins of the same size when using them for storage, as these will stack better and take up less room.
- Using vacuum pack bags for clothing, bedding, etc., is an excellent option as these can easily slide under beds or be placed on top of cupboards for easy access instead of being stored in a bin.
- Storage ottomans can also provide additional seating in the lounge and are perfect for storing books, games, and technology paraphernalia for gaming.

Remember, it's not how big the house is, but how happy the home is.

Identifying Communal Time and Spaces

Living together again in a shared space will present interesting challenges, including sharing areas such as lounges and bathrooms; sharing bathrooms has always created drama in many households, and ideally, it would be perfect if, as adults, you did not have to do this. But your circumstances may not allow for this, so a clear and reasonable structure must be agreed upon to prevent bathroom wars and dramas. Cleaning up behind yourself is another common cause of family squabbles, and this has to be addressed as no one wants to feel that they are doing more than their fair share, nor should you be cleaning up after your adult child anyway.

Certain times of the day could be set aside for communal living in a specific area that is acceptable to everyone. Voicing the reasoning of why these times have been chosen can be presented and why this area might be off-limits at certain times.

Whatever results you come up with regarding communal spaces, it is critical to be clear about the dos and don'ts so that everyone in the household is on the same page. This communication will ensure clarity and help make everyone feel comfortable that they are acting within the set parameters.

This could also involve setting expectations regarding each other's visitors and the parameters. It is more than acceptable to understand that your adult children might not want you involved in their friend's visits and need a bit of private space and just space to have their conversations without mom and dad. Being reasonable and finding a way to give your adult children privacy in your home is possible. It just takes a bit of juggling around. The main thing is to be clear that no one is continuously being compromised of their own space.

Setting the Ground Rules for Living Together

With any situation, be it a work environment or a home one, there has to be a set of ground rules that everyone is aware of to ensure a smooth outcome. How are you meant to understand or know if you have not been made aware of a required behavior or structure?

Finding the balance of what works is different for everyone, and there are no set hard and fast rules of what will work for every household. For instance, perhaps one family member loves to cook and wants to be responsible for cooking all the meals but does not want to do any laundry. You will have to find what ground rules work for your household and what is required to keep it fair and balanced.

The predominant factor here is that this is a household of adults where the responsibilities of cohabitation should be shared —being practical about the day-to-day struggle of chores that nobody wants to do can be significantly reduced when they are shared. In particular, those thankless household tasks of laundry, taking out the trash, cleaning, etc. Finding the advantage in negative situations is quite enlightening when you realize you have another set of responsible hands to lighten your load!

Although your adult child will be living at home, this is not an opening for the parents to continuously fix their problems while living together. If they persist in wanting you to sort out their issues without any attempt to try on their own, this should become part of the ground rules for yourself to acknowledge. Rather than jumping in to fix whatever has cropped up, relay your faith in them and highlight their abilities that they may be doubting. Discussing in-depth the available resources and support structure they have, including all their available options, will start the process. Reaffirm their skills and intelligence to find the solution with some logically based thinking. Explaining that sometimes just talking through a problem with you or a friend can bring the answer for themselves without you taking it on to resolve it.

All of this will take some tolerance and an acceptance of being reasonable about the effects of living together. Make sure that these ground rules being established are not only for the nitty-gritty of daily life but also a platform to help your adult children stand on their own two feet with a good support structure until they can do it alone.

Setting Expectations

The defined clarity of what your expectations are is necessary here. Being vague about your needs and then being upset when they are not met with what was going on in your head is unfair to anyone and can cause unnecessary upsets for everyone involved.

If you make a habit of ignoring the ground rules set and letting things slide when they are broken, it may contribute to a negative relationship as there are no clear guidelines. It undermines the point of establishing some ground rules in the first place. This could result in your adult child not taking any responsibility for themselves as you are a softie who will just give in if they bat their eyelids or give you that sweet smile. It is a form of manipulation, and giving in just does not help them one little bit. It will only contribute to your adult child having an unrealistic expectation that you will sort it out and let them off this time and the next, so it continues into a downward spiral.

Perhaps, when your children were growing up, you hung out the washing in the lounge as it may have had a nice sunny spot in winter. Your adult comes home years later and does the same thing, thinking it is okay and cannot understand why it is not. They may be confused about your reaction as you may not have mentioned that it is something you do not do anymore. It might all sound a little silly, but it is often the little things that are left unsaid that are the ones that can become significant problems.

Depending on what your household has agreed upon, the best time is to have the weekly *pow-wow* with each other; it is the opportunity to bring up any issues that need to be dealt with. Nipping things in the bud as they happen can often not be the right time. If everyone meets together regularly at family dinner time, that can be the best time to discuss how things are going informally. Trying to deal with an issue when everyone is rushing around to leave for work in the morning causes undue stress and a poor outcome. Choose your time wisely to deal with and voice your expectations. Just be sure to deal with any ground rules that have been adhered to and not let them slip away with a view of it being too late now to deal with them.

If your adult child has ignored a non-negotiable, being very clear about second chances, if you decide that the transgression is worthy of it, it should probably be dealt with immediately rather than leaving it to annoy you until the family meeting. There must be clear consequences for not following house rules; otherwise, why have them at all? Establishing these rules together will give everyone in the household some ownership of them and should ultimately ensure that they are followed. Being part of the process of setting boundaries will solve half of the problem as all would have had an opportunity to have their say and find a workable solution.

This is all about finding the balance between what works for your household; again, it must be reiterated that there are no hard-set rules that work for everyone. Every family differs from the next, depending on religion, culture, and values. Only you can decide what will work to maintain harmony in the home.

6

YOUR NEW ADULT–ADULT RELATIONSHIP

Families are the compass that guides us. They are the inspiration to reach great heights and our comfort when we occasionally falter. –Brad Henry

It is a huge blessing when a parent reaches the stage of being a parent to an adult child. Reaching this period of your life can be the most rewarding time for both of you. It can also be challenging, as you will need to work on understanding how your relationship has evolved. When your adult child moves back home, this places even more emphasis on this. They are not returning as a child, and probably the closest way to describe this is that it is almost as if they are returning as a guest in your home. Making anyone, whoever they are, feel welcome and comfortable when they stay in your home appeals to just about everybody, so why would you want it another way?

It can catch us off guard when our adult children live with us, as we might find ourselves falling back into the *over-parenting* role without even noticing it. We simply may not have moved through the parenting stage and need a reminder to do it; otherwise, there may be some adverse effects in your relationship being caused by it.

THE STAGES OF GROWTH

There are some defined stages of parenting that are split into a few stages that we sometimes get stuck in. Dividing these stages into age groups is probably the easiest way to explain this process. I am sure you will relate to a great deal of the information compiled about these stages for some context from babyhood to adulthood.

- Birth to 5 years

Becoming a parent is a big adjustment you can only understand once you have become one. During this stage, the parent's role can be described as a commander or a caregiver. You are on duty 24/7 with the loving, nurturing, feeding, caring, and constantly watching over them. You essentially do everything for your child and also teach them and tell them what they can and cannot do, sometimes with reasons and sometimes with none. It is an exhausting but exhilarating time when the parents grow up very fast, realizing that this child is dependent on you for survival. This time in your child's life culminates with them starting to take their first baby steps in becoming independent with the start of their school phase.

- 5 to 12 years

A coach or trainer is probably the closest description to your role during this stage. They are becoming more independent and are beginning to understand themselves a bit more, which will show in their behavior. Your role will be to help teach them how to be more responsible as they will have so many choices presented to them during the early years of schooling without you being there every step of the way. Being involved in their lives and helping them make good decisions is very important during these foundation years of schooling. It can be quite an emotional time for the parent to see the babyhood disappear and perhaps even start to see a bit of themselves in their children's behaviors.

- 12 to 18 years

A parent of a teenager has a redefined role in their lives, and an advisor or counselor would best describe this. At this stage of their lives, it is a massive step for parents to accept that they are no longer the primary influencer in their child's life. Your children are stepping away from being reliant on you for decisions or opinions and are determined to make their own way.

Be consistent in your encouragement, and support, and allow them to grow with the confidence that you have instilled a good foundation of values in their pre-teen years. Always making the decisions for your teenager will just hinder their step into adulthood, particularly if they are not allowed to suffer the consequences of poor choices that they may make. Rebelling against structures, rules, and parents is quite common during the teenage years. Additionally, dealing with hormonal changes adds to some of the conflicts during these years, considered by most parents to be the most challenging!

- Over 18 years

And finally, we reach adulthood, where the parent and the child reach friendship. The parents have a big job of letting go and almost assuming the role of becoming a consultant in their adult child's life. How the process has unfolded in the previous stages creates the foundation for what comes next. Be available to your child for support, be involved but not over-involved, and do a lot of letting go!

This is not a perfect science, as we all have different personalities and circumstances that will determine how these stages unfold and when they will overlap. These stages have been outlined for you to refer to and reflect on the different times of your child's life and how your behavior was at that time. It could help clarify some difficulties you may encounter while having your adult child at home by chatting about their childhood and mistakes that were perhaps made along the way. No parent is perfect, and ownership of mistakes and how they are dealt with together with our children is what makes a family function.

Confession time! Having not progressed fully into the realization that I should be in the role of a consultant, I slipped into the previous roles of caregiver, coach, and counselor. It would be with the stark realization that I had to face up to the fact that I had not grown, and they had. It was time for me to do some growing of my own. Motherhood was the most enjoyable time and being presented with this opportunity to *mother* them again came all too easily.

I had not adequately prepared for this stage and had not read anything to make me wiser! It is pretty freeing to let go of this responsibility and adopt the role of consultant with your adult children asking for advice when they need it.

LEARNING HOW NOT TO MICROMANAGE

As a parent of this person who now lives in your home, it may be difficult not to over-parent them. For some parents, learning the art of not micromanaging their adult child living under their roof is a considerable challenge.

Those parental instincts and control you had when they were

children do not disappear overnight; it is a process. Learning to control the urge not to advise your adult children unless they ask for it is quite a hard lesson to learn. If they have not asked for your advice, hold it back for when they do. Constantly pushing advice and your words of wisdom, even if it is coming from a good place, can create an outcome of them just eventually not sharing what is going on in their lives. This goes for all sorts of things, from exercise, decor, health, food, and so on. It may not be the appropriate time for you to give your input. Be very aware of this letting-go phase.

Imagine if every time you had an idea or something you were considering and just wanted to share your thoughts but were met with a barrage of advice, be it negative or positive. You would be irritated. Thinking of establishing your new role as a parent and now switching to a consultant will be a productive process. It seems a little business-like, but it is probably the closest thing to beginning to understand your new role, particularly if your adult children are in a relationship. This adds another angle as they probably bounce ideas off their partner and would expect their advice, similar to you and your partner or spouse when you discuss ideas together. Be willing to allow them the respect and freedom an adult rightly deserves in their relationships without being overbearing and controlling. Think of your new role as a sounding board for them, and work hard to break down old habits of telling them what to do. Just listen. Find the positive in adverse situations by doing your utmost not to be critical of their decisions and being able to encourage them to follow their instincts. Creating a relationship that is always open and honest, without a barrage of advice, will pave the way for them to return to you for advice when they need it.

Becoming an adult is the start of independence, which is already being compromised for them by needing to move back home. Do not drown them in your *expert advice* unless asked for it.

Squelch it. Your adult child deserves trust and the opportunity to find their path. Give them the space and the grace to do so.

What you do need to do is to communicate with them fairly and clearly about what your concerns are. Talking about transgressions causing problems is required to find the solutions to move forward together and maintain a happy household. You are aiming to find and solve these issues together as consenting adults.

Setting Healthy Relationship Boundaries

Acceptance of letting go of the way of thinking that you always know what is best for them is essential in creating healthy relationship boundaries. The same would apply to your adult child, too, with not expecting mom and dad to sort out their problems. The need to participate in each other's lives in a supportive role without controlling the situation is the aim. Be involved but not over-involved in each other's lives. Care, trust, and respect for each other are integral to having a solid parent and adult-child relationship. This ensures that neither party is crowding the others' space and that the freedom that each one deserves is respected.

Never underestimate the importance of the need for support your adult child may require from time to time when they ask for it. Adult children also need to understand that sometimes their parents are not in a position to help them due to circumstances that might stop them from doing whatever they may have been asked to do. Nurturing your relationship with the love and support of each other constantly will ground all of you to know that you are always there for each other no matter what and no matter the circumstances. Sometimes it is just a hug that is needed. No words, no money, no stuff—just a hug. Gentle love and support are sometimes the only things that are needed.

If there is a blatant disregard for each other's need for independence and when respect is put aside, this can cause long-lasting damage to your relationships. Emotional distress and the anxiety of feeling unsupported and not acknowledged are detrimental and very hard to fix.

Make time for each other, not only to sort out problems but also to have fun. Spending quality, happy time together is like the glue for love that keeps families unified. Remember that they also have their lives and probably do not want to spend all their free time with you. Again, find the balance. Try not to be disappointed if they choose to do something else with their friends instead of you, as long as this has been done respectfully. This means that it is not okay if they have arranged to do something with you as a family and then drop you to instead spend time with their friends without any thought of how this could upset you.

Having healthy relationships also involves how much financial aid you give. Suppose you consistently give your adult child money or keep paying for things they can ill afford. In that case, you could create a big problem of unhealthy relationship boundaries regarding financial issues. You will know better from experience how much you value an item you have saved and paid for. By continuously giving, you are blurring the boundaries for your adult child to gain this feeling of self-worth and value. There is, of course, the reasoning that you want to make things easier for your children than perhaps you experienced, but in the end, this just short-changes them in realizing these boundaries have been set to be adhered to and not to be blurry when it suits them.

Communicate regularly with them about valuing what you have paid for to inspire them to choose what is essential and what is a need and not a want—even if it means they experience some hardships along the way. Financial issues with your adult child can cause strife in your relationship with each other, so being sure you have relayed your boundaries about any funds involved between you is crucial. Whether it is a loan, gift, some bridging finance, paying off a debt, or whatever the reason is, ensuring everyone understands and accepts the criteria will help keep your relationship healthy.

Your relationship with each other is not about money. It is about love and support that should be consistent in their lives from you.

Everyone deserves the freedom to choose what they want to do as long as it is done maturely and respectfully, which does not cause someone to be intentionally hurt by those actions. Similarly, if someone is unintentionally hurt by actions taken, this must be addressed, and responsibility must be taken to repair the hurt feelings. Owning up and dealing with mistakes is integral for both sides of the parent and adult child relationship to take it to a new and mutually supportive role.

7

FINDING YOUR PEACE

Take the opportunity to learn from your mistakes; find the cause of your problems and eliminate it. Don't try to be perfect; just try to be an excellent example of being human. –Tony Robbins

This could be a time of your life when you and your spouse or partner have settled into an easy, comfortable rhythm without having children in the house. All those years of child-rearing and caring for a family can sometimes be tough on a marriage. The commitment you have as parents never ease off during these years. No matter how your family was brought up, be it by one of the parents staying at home or working and carers being involved, our dynamics are all different. The one thing that is the same is that you are parents for life, no matter what. When your children finally reach adulthood and move out, there is a definite change in the relationship with your spouse or partner that will also take time to adapt. Realizations and affirmations to each other are another whole new stage of your relationship. It is also a time of finding your new balance with each other and exploring life differently without children. Some couples have never been together without children. So, this can be a brand-new or whimsical look into the past before children came along. Whatever the circumstances, even if you are single and have created a life of your own, things will change quite a bit.

An adult child coming home to live under your roof once again can cause this balance to be unsettled and enhance it to be an even more blissful time. When a household is full of adults, a benefit is that the responsibilities should be shared, which can create some extra downtime for all. Leave everyone with more time to choose to do what fulfills them and gives them their inner peace.

The home environment you created before they moved back in must still suit you. Any changes you might have to adapt to with this change of circumstances need to be agreed on by everyone involved, regardless of the living situation.

If there is strife and anguish stemming from the move of your adult child coming back home, and if it is not dealt with appropriately, it will only cause less peace and more difficulties. Be focused on the situation at hand and the acceptance that everyone in the household is in this together to make it work. The support structure will benefit everyone if all parties are ready to take responsibility for their actions.

In the previous chapter, we mentioned that you should own up to your mistakes and rectify them with appropriate measures. This certainly applies to keeping the peace when you do this. It does not have to be a whole heavy and intense meeting with each other. It could be a walk and then a gentle touch on a shoulder and apologizing for placing them in a difficult position or situation and how sorry you are for hurting their feelings.

Meaningful apologies can mend relationships with a cement-like type of glue of love. Being sincere and not flippant about behaviors will teach your adult children to value genuine apologies. In turn, they will be able to mirror this behavior of apologizing when they are in a similar situation. Apologies are challenging to appreciate if the person apologizes to you and then adds on a *but* at the end of it, which in a sense is a way of validating their poor behavior and placing blame on the person who needs the apology. This is not an apology; it is wanting to be excused for bad behavior and not taking responsibility for inappropriate actions.

If you find yourselves in a situation where a big rift is forming, consider these actions to address them peacefully.

- Be the one who steps forward to initiate the changes needed with the focus on what this change needs to be instead of who was right and who was wrong. If blaming each other is the focus, it could lead to an even bigger rift.
- Ditch the silent treatment as it most often builds up resentment, and even though the surroundings may be quieter, it is certainly not helpful in trying to find your peace. Think of silence before the storm brewing.
- Be careful with hurtful words that can create deep, lasting damage. It happens to everyone, and we have all been guilty of it, where something is said in anger and not meant. Tackle this head-on to apologize profusely and meaningfully to the person you hurt, even if it means writing a note to explain yourself clearly. Be brave and stand up and deal with something you have done wrong.
- Be humble in your approach, do your utmost not to control a situation, and allow others to give their input to resolve it. Acceptance that you do not always know best is a big step to take in humility. Sometimes, we overstep our boundaries without even noticing. Consider a trigger word agreed on in the family that will jolt anyone stepping out of line and reconsider their actions. We use *Brussels sprouts* as our trigger word to help

maintain the peace. A note of caution is not to use this trigger word jokingly as it will lose its powerfulness in potentially soothing a volatile situation.

- Find a neutral space to have difficult discussions where everyone feels equal. This could be a coffee shop or a bench under a tree. Taking conversations away from the home where it was more than likely to be the place where the rift was started really helps. This is mainly because it is your home and not theirs anymore, so they may feel insecure when trying to deal with something big under your roof. It gives a fresh perspective on situations too.
- Even when things are tense, being told that you are loved and that you matter will help ease the tension. We all thrive on being nurtured and loved. Telling each other, often and with meaning, that they are loved is the foundation for mutual support. Take a moment to face each other and be sincere about your words.
- Acceptance that perhaps this situation cannot be mended in one session and that more time is needed. If this happens and a resolution cannot be agreed upon or reached, that is also okay. What is not okay is to leave the situation unresolved. If you cannot resolve it at the end of your discussion, then agree to pick it up again at another time. Being consistent in the completion of finding an acceptable result is a good value to instill, not only for disagreements but ultimately for everything in life. Finish what you start. Patience and care are closely related words to creating peaceful outcomes.

These suggestions listed above could also be helpful by sharing them with your adult child. Having them contribute to what they perceive as a productive method to restore peace in the home will be constructive for them. It should also help make them feel included in a process important to keep the peace. Everyone wants a peaceful life and to be happy. Learning how to develop it takes practice.

My deep spiritual connection with God gave me a sense of peace. Finding my peace was by having quiet moments in the mornings with my God.

"Better a dry crust with peace and quiet, than a full house full of feasting with strife" (*The Holy Bible, New International Version*, 1973/2011, Proverbs 17:1).

Sometimes, doing a yoga session or walking would also help me find my perspective and make everything seem much clearer. My husband is not good at managing conflict, as he is a natural peacemaker. Whenever a situation arose where he felt flustered, he would give me *that look* that I know so well and say he was off for a walk. I knew he needed time and space to gather his thoughts and gain perspective on whatever was bothering him.

I felt strongly about creating fun times together with the family and encouraged all of us to be able to laugh. We would often exercise together by playing a tennis match, going for walks, or doing yoga in the lounge.

We would often end up in fits of laughter stemming from the fierce but friendly competition when playing board games over a good couple of glasses of wine. This brings back such fond memories of our special time together. Other events we enjoyed that were planned together were a mid-winter Christmas dinner decked with all the trimmings to make it feel like December. We also had pizza evenings and prosecco nights and even created some hilarious TikTok dances together, which are priceless to watch now. These are treasured and unforgettable memories for all of us.

AVOIDING THOSE NEGATIVE FEELINGS

It is hard for parents to break the habit of being the carer, the sorter-outer, and ultimately, the one that deals with their child's problems. The key word in that sentence is *child*. They are no longer a child but adults; even though they live under your roof, they need to deal with the issues and circumstances they find themselves in as adults.

It can be upsetting for a parent whose adult child is struggling to make ends meet or to establish themselves independently. Identifying each other's roles on the homefront can help when the future is a bit uncertain. Having stability and clarity in one spectrum of anyone's life does help pave the way for other things to fall into place. When everything is haphazard and disorganized with no structure, this can lead to a feeling of negativity and a bleak view of one's self-worth. Be careful and do your utmost to avoid falling into the pit of negative emotions.

For those susceptible to depression, in the case of either parent or adult children, this change of circumstances can be hard to deal with until the balance is created. Positive reinforcement and emotional support are crucial. Never be afraid to ask for help; know that it is a sign of strength, not weakness, when you ask for it.

There could be a flurry of emotions you need to deal with, from confusion, frustration, guilt, irritation, relief, sadness, and happiness in the early days of this new phase. Focus on the good, and let the negative feelings go. Give yourself time to adapt and embrace it all. There is no quick-fix solution but only guidelines to help the process be less stressful. If your adult child is driving you up the wall, deal with it positively with a solution or an alternative to consider (instead of just focusing on the negative).

On both sides, everyone should be aware of their power of choice to choose not to engage in negativity and conflict, and this should be respected. You are all adults in this and are entitled to make your own decisions, bearing in mind that this must not negatively impact anyone. Avoiding negative situations is not to be used as an excuse not to deal with problems. Try to have empathy and put yourself in the other person's shoes; this is often the way forward.

Creating Your Personal Alone Time

This is one of the most important words of advice to give you. The well-being of your mental health is essential, and to have some alone time without being the parent or even your spouse, for that matter, is good for you. As a parent with adult children, you have reached the stage where it is more than justified for some well-earned personal alone time, and it is necessary. Whatever fulfills you to achieve that sense of equilibrium in your life, do it. Do not ever feel guilty about taking some time out for yourself.

Sometimes, adult children's expectations of their parents need some adjusting. They will have to accept that their parents will not be at their beck and call for everything. Falling back into old patterns they were used to as children is unacceptable. This is not only for physical help with certain things but even more so for emotional and financial support. If your adult child insists on crowding your personal alone time with their needs, make them aware you are entitled to time alone. They might be blissfully unaware of the intrusion and may need to be told to give you your space. Explaining the importance of this time for you and its benefits to your mental health should set the record straight with them. At the same time, they would perhaps realize and acknowledge their selfishness in their expectations of you always being there for them. It also would hopefully have an effect on them making a similar choice for themselves and taking out some personal time alone if they are not accustomed to doing so already.

Creating Space for Your Relationship

At this stage of your life, you and your partner/spouse may have begun to find your newly established balance with each other without the children around. It is a critical time for both of you and must not be compromised by the advent of your adult children moving back home. Working on your relationship to make time for yourselves to focus on your needs, not those of your adult child, is very necessary. There is nothing wrong with focusing on yourselves and not your adult children.

When your adult children have left home, you get a new opportunity to discover your relationship as a couple and recharge the romance back into your lives, especially if it was waning a bit! It is also a time to hone your friendship with each other again, without all the responsibilities you had together as parents. Tweaking those memories of what attracted you to each other and why you are together sometimes needs a bit of re-evaluation. It may have been a very long time since you have been alone together and are enjoying this new relationship with each other.

When adult children move back in, you need to be fully aware that this does not negatively impact your relationship with each other. It will be new for everyone as expectations of the same behaviors are a common occurrence. When these behaviors or reactions are different, this can cause some upheaval and misunderstandings for everyone involved. Some will struggle to adapt to these changes, especially if they have not been communicated beforehand. For example, if the mother of the household always used to take care of all the laundry with no questions asked, and perhaps now, when the adult child is back home, they think this would be the same. Maybe it is now the dad that does it, and the mom does not lift a finger with the laundry. Adult children may be puzzled why mom is not doing their laundry anymore, or hopefully, they will be doing it without being asked to do it anyway!

This is a very simple example but should give you an idea and a pause for thought on how many things you *usually did* as a parent of children and no longer do anymore. Discussing these different things with your partner or spouse and deciding what is good for you as a couple and what is not is a good process to go through with each other.

There will be more challenges faced when wanting to do something spontaneous, and you will need to figure out how not to lose this fun aspect of having a good relationship with each other. By this stage of your marriage, you are both well aware of the work it takes to have a solid relationship! Keeping the love alive and not stopping things like date night just because your adult child is now at home is important. Probably, the newfound love you have for each other will inspire and motivate your adult child to get their life together and find what you have for themselves too.

8

COUNTING YOUR BLESSINGS

This is part of what a family is about, not just love. It's knowing that your family will be there watching out for you. Nothing else will give you that. Not money. Not fame. Not work. –Mitch Albom

This situation of your adult child coming home for a while would likely not be permanent and will be as temporary as you both negotiate and agree on a time frame. This will be based on what parameters have been set and agreed upon. Family is so important, and support for each other has no price tag and should be nurtured. It cannot be measured in monetary wealth or the possessions you have. How do you place a value on love?

It can be the most wonderful time in your lives, as you will be establishing a whole new relationship together based on the maturity and support of each other. The relatable things you will have in common now are numerous, providing an exciting and wonderful platform to explore together. Establishing this mature and new relationship with each other will open doors to other parts of your lives that you may not have been aware of. There will be things to discover that you both enjoy and can relate to. Overall, there are far more positives to experience than negatives. Perhaps in the past, the teenage years were a bit rocky and caused many upheavals, whereas now, as adults, it is easier to communicate your needs without those raging hormones getting in the way! Appreciate your precious time together and do not sweat the small stuff. There is always a way to find a resolution to a problem.

For the adult child, it is a window of opportunity for them to hit pause and reset, to figure out their intended and realistic goals and how they can best achieve them with some financial and emotional support from their parents. Taking advice from parents is sometimes not easy for adult children to do as they want to make their own decisions. Something that should be mentioned is that if the parents are funding specific projects, their adult children must count their blessings too and be willing to involve their parents in those decisions they are making when spending these funds. If the parents can offer this window of opportunity to their child and then witness their adult child progressing through this stage, it can be a sublime experience. It is almost like a newfound connection being offered to be with your child and being able to venture into a new journey together.

The appreciation and joy I have for the time we were given to spend together and the shared moments would not have been possible without this experience. Having adult children back in your home creates many opportunities to bring awareness of different perspectives into your life on subjects from politics and current affairs to general life.

Our discussions around the dinner table as adults were a platform for many meaningful and richly rewarding conversations ranging from climate change and our different views on it to implementing minimalism into your life.

The blessing of sharing in the accomplishments of your adult children's goals when they reach them is priceless. There are also those incredible moments that probably would not have been shared if they had not lived at home at the time. In particular, we felt very privileged that one of our adult children confided in us about a deeply personal struggle they were experiencing. Because of this, we were able to offer support and love.

APPRECIATING THIS TIME

The time you have been given to reconnect with your adult child is a gift and should not be undermined by any negative issues. Working through these negatives together can give your adult-to-adult relationship new meaning. The younger generation's insight about dealing with conflict will sometimes surprise you. The world they have grown up in is quite different from when you were growing up, so their insight can be mutually beneficial.

Having a peek into their adult world, and seeing how they are adapting and growing up, can be an illuminating experience as they achieve their goals. Reconnecting with each other, understanding, and accepting how to offer your advice, is easier to do living together than apart.

Your adult child will flourish in the support and care you can offer them, while your focus is not to be overpowering or manipulating their decisions to what you think is best. Encourage them to dive deep into themselves to begin to gain an understanding that they do know what is best for them. Make sure that they know you are here to help guide them if they ask for it. Break those barriers of mistrust and aggression, and find the ultimate way forward that makes them feel like adults, not co-dependent children. Developing these key areas will broaden the foundation of your relationship with your adult children, where they will feel confident in approaching you for assistance without feelings of judgment or ridicule. Ask your adult children about their lives and focus on showing you are curious about their visions for their future and not questioning their decision or wanting to meddle in their affairs. Talk about real stuff, what makes them happy or sad, what inspires them, and what they dream about and yearn for. Maybe consider forming new and improved family traditions with their input into what they feel would be beneficial. Creating these special family times with their input will bring a fresh perspective to family gatherings. Perhaps you may reinforce old traditions or let them go to make way for something new.

Try not to forget the importance of grabbing every single opportunity to have fun together and do things that you love with each other—doing projects together as adults are quite different from when they were children. You may be pleasantly amazed and surprised at what they can offer in newfound skills they have that you may not be aware of. It is about making every moment count and sharing the responsibilities that life throws at us. It is an unbelievably special time for parents and adult children that does not happen for everyone.

There is this to keep in mind: According to research done about boomerang children, it is said that years later, adult children are more likely to care for parents who helped them during the tough times (Kennedy & Farrell, 2019). Some food for thought, but of course, not to be the motivation behind allowing them to come live with you. Some conditions like this might be viewed as offensive or too conditional.

Taking the Time to Be Together

The undeniable advantage of living together is all the extra face-to-face time you have with each other. When they get on with their lives and move out, these times spent together become less. Using this extra time you have to create a deeper bond with each other should not go amiss. Try to set aside some alone time with your adult child; the value of a one-on-one session is immeasurable.

Bouncing ideas off each other can be fun and can also be

enlightening to discover how great the advice is that your adult child could offer you. If they have been out of the home for some time before moving back in, some of the lessons and life skills they have learned may surprise you. Giving them this opportunity of being the one who provides advice instead of the other way around states that you are accepting them as an equal, an adult, and not a child anymore. It is a marvelous bonding time! Perhaps, redecorating the house and modernizing it may be appealing and needed. Go shopping together and value their input instead of sticking to what you have always bought.

Share special times, attend live music festivals and events, dress up and dance the night away together, and have fun. Perhaps, watch sports events that you both enjoy or even one you know nothing about but is their passion. This opens up more opportunities for your adult child to share their interests and teach you something you did not know much about. If you are feeling brave, perhaps try out an activity you might never have considered doing before with them. Taking the plunge and doing something you have never done before can be exhilarating and creates eternal memories.

Family trips together as adults are quite different from the "Are we there yet?" trips when they were young children. It does not have to be a luxurious holiday. It could be a trip with no destination too! Finding new areas to explore together and going on walking, fishing, or cycling adventures can be enriching. Adding in experiences, like wine tasting and food pairing, that can be enjoyed together now as adults can stimulate new interests together.

Find ways to make the usual household chores fun, experience new cooking methods, and do it together. Blind tasting competitions are great fun if enthusiastic cooks are in the house. There are so many volunteering opportunities you might be interested in doing together to add some meaningfulness to others who need it when spending your time together.

Take trips down memory lane together and sort through old photos that perhaps your adult child can help you digitize. Find those old videos and do the same. Enjoying old home movies together and sharing those special memories is a joy. Connecting again with family members you might not have seen in a while is also something good to do as adults, particularly if they have not seen them since they were a child. Nurturing the bonds with other family members and keeping these connections alive can benefit you and them.

If they are in a relationship, take the time to get to know their partner but take care not to meddle in their relationship. Let them be the guide of how involved you can be, as this is a personal relationship they are building, and they might not want your involvement. You need to respect that.

Whatever you choose to do together and how you spend your time, the emphasis is on quality time together and making these special moments count. If you are a writer, you could even journal these moments you are experiencing with them and perhaps give them this journal a few years later.

Treating Them Like an Adult

There is nothing worse than an adult child being treated like a child. Even though the decision to move back home was theirs, it should not be treated as a failure. If you think like this, your attitude may need to be adjusted, as this could create discontentment and harm your relationship.

Positive affirmation will go a long way. Some parents may worry about what their circle of friends may think about it and perhaps are fearful of judgment too. This should be the least of your concerns. Besides, there are probably many parents that would love to have their adult children home for a while and might be green with envy that you are fortunate to have this time together—never mind also taking a moment to acknowledge that your children like you enough to want to come home!

It is also a time to ensure that your adult child feels supported and cared for. However, you want to avoid them becoming codependent on you or for them to regress to their childhood behaviors.

The emphasis is on how your language is presented when your adult child is doing something you do not entirely agree upon. Telling anyone they are wrong, in most cases, immediately causes a feeling of resentment. Instead, approach the given situation with alternatives to dealing with that particular occurrence. Presenting an abrupt or an outright *no* may raise some hackles!

There are also instances of too much teasing or guilt shaming in these circumstances that are harmful and not helpful. Using basic logic and approaching your adult child with reasonable observations and suggestions is ample to change the outcome without raising any feeling of hurt or resentment.

Be aware of your adult child becoming depressed as this situation they are in might result in a negative impact on them. This could occur if their envisaged plans are not coming to fruition and some factors are out of their control. They might feel a bit of a downward spiral, unable to see a way out, and feel like a burden to you. As their parents, you are the most crucial support structure they have. Discussing these problematic issues as adults and ensuring them of your emotional support and help, and always being there for them, can help with depression. Watch out for severe depression and anxiety and if they need professional help, be gentle with persuading them to seek the help they need with your support.

Alongside treating your adult children as adults comes the necessity to not give up the essential things in your life that you were participating in before they moved back in. You have parented them as children and are long past the stage of having to be home to ensure dinner is on the table. They are responsible adults now and can think and care for themselves too. Maintaining your social life and hobbies is very important to keep up with you and your partner or spouse, as your life should not stop because your adult children have moved back home. Keeping things simple, by perhaps agreeing to dinner together one evening every week and leaving the rest of the week flexible, suits some families. Having adult conversations with your children can be delightful and educational too!

Finding what works for your household of adults together can be enjoyable and not demanding. Keep in mind that this living situation is new and different and that it is a household of adults who all have opinions that matter.

9

EXECUTING THE EXIT PLAN

I've learned that people will forget what you said, people will forget what you did, but people will never forget how you made them feel.
–Maya Angelou

In most circumstances, adult children moving back home will usually be a short-term plan as there are not many adult children who would choose to live with their parents indefinitely, and vice versa! The empty nest period, although sometimes a bit of a sad time to see your children leave the nest, also has fabulous appeal to parents. This is a special time that ideally does not feel like a burden, as it is also an opportunity to reconnect with your adult children. Be mindful that you put extra effort into the relationship with your spouse, ensuring this does not diminish at this time. We all know having children is a lifetime commitment, but some freedom is expected when they become adults. As much as we love them, we need our time too! Making sure you have a clear exit plan that has been discussed with your adult child before moving in is sound advice.

When you were first approached about them moving in, a

discussion should have been held about how long it would be. Emphasis is placed on the exit plan being formulated to help them gain their independence once more and not to be a case of throwing them out. Just as in nature, baby birds cannot stay in the nest forever.

Once your adult child has a clear strategy of their goals for the next few weeks, months, and years, this process will be much smoother. As discussed in the book, goals can be adapted depending on circumstances, but the importance of having some goals is something to be acknowledged. Helping your adult child to keep on track with their goals and allowing them to make the changes when they need to be adapted is essential. It does not help them if you lay out the entire plan and tell them what to do. They will have a hard time adjusting to your plan if they have not had any input. The key is guidance. Regular checking in with them to see where they are with their goal plan is strongly advised while they are living with you, so you are kept in the loop with their progress. Again, it is an advisory role, not a micromanaging one.

HAVING THE NECESSARY TIMELINE DISCUSSION

When discussing timelines, part of this conversation could include how to secure a job that has stability for them. A position with benefits is a bonus! Establish a realistic budget to look at for finding a place of their own to move into eventually. This budget is essential as it will clearly indicate what they need to save—to pay for the deposit required and to start building up a nest egg for those never-ending incidentals. There are always hidden costs when moving into a new place; perhaps now is the time to take this opportunity to think of what these could be. Simple things like when starting fresh and moving into a brand-new place, the food bill will be significantly higher to start with as you would not have essential pantry items like spices, oil, sauces, etc., that you would not necessarily buy each time you shop. A great idea is to consider having a pantry party for them before they move out. Friends and family can be involved and help contribute to these basics to give them a practical helping hand to get started. This will ease the burden off them of those expensive setup costs, and everyone will feel they have played a part in contributing to helping effectively.

When having timeline discussions, much will depend on how long you have agreed for them to live with you, as this will determine the planning strategy. If it is months, for example, then work in perhaps six-week periods to achieve certain steps towards the goal. Not having a plan or a timeline framework for building up to the exit date leaves no clear way forward to set goals and achieve objectives that need to be reached for them to gain their independence. Even if they do not know how long it will take for them to reach the stage of moving out, then perhaps consider breaking it up into three-month re-evaluation stages if this suits you.

Strategizing the Exit

Ensuring the process has some clear guidelines to work within helps achieve a smooth outcome without drama and angst. The overwhelming need parents have to only want what is best for their children, even when they are adults, never goes away!

Choosing what you can provide to help ease their battle for independence depends on your circumstances as to what can be offered when setting out the strategy for their exit plan. The key is to be mutually respectful with each other no matter what the eventual plan is going to be. Here are some guidelines to help you formulate a strategy that will work for your household.

1. Ensure you and your partner or spouse agree on what decisions have been made.

Apart from wanting to ensure your adult children's happiness and independence, if this is overlooked, it can cause undue stress and potential damage to your relationship. Agreeing on the broad outline of your expectations and goals, and finding the middle ground that works for both of you is crucial for the health of your relationship. At the end of the day, you both will be worse off if you have not communicated your needs with each other. Sometimes, even counseling is suggested if the situation of your adult children causes undue stress and upset in your relationship. Taking sides never works, and neither does keeping secrets from each other.

2. Be clear about what you can and cannot provide.

When you are being vague or unclear about what you can provide in terms of support both during and after your adult children move out, it can cause confusion for them. In today's world, many families struggle to handle the stresses of the poor economic situation affecting most of us. Being able to pull together and support each other realistically with what you can offer is critical. Chances of building up resentment if you have overcompensated in one sphere are unpleasant and could potentially damage relationships. Sometimes, the best lessons we learn are the ones that make us hit rock bottom, so also be aware of allowing your adult children to make their own mistakes and deal with the consequences.

3. Maintain respectful behavior even when things go wrong.

You may have created the perfect plan on paper, yet in reality, it might not work. Never be afraid to admit it when you are wrong, as this in turn teaches your adult child the same behavior. As parents, allowing our adult children to accept responsibility is a huge part of growing up and being independent. Focus on achieving the stages that are needed to eventually lead to implementing the exit plan, and be prepared to probably have to adjust things without derailing the outcome with negative behaviors. Being clear that eventually, they will need to move out even if the timelines are changed is important and not an excuse to keep extending the date.

4. Stop the guilty payments.

In some situations, adult children may continue to expect their parents to keep bailing them out of tough financial situations. It is hard to say no to someone you love and want to help, but continuously enabling them to use you as a symbolic ATM, is not okay. Your strategy plan leading up to them moving out includes cutting those purse strings. There will always be differences and as hard as we try not to do it, we do judge each other. For example, if your adult child suddenly purchases an unnecessarily expensive vehicle instead of paying the deposit for their flat and now wants to extend their stay with you and change the strategy of your exit plan you have agreed upon. On the other hand, you could have purchased something expensive, and your adult child is resentful and intimates you should have instead spent it on their flat deposit. These alternative examples of circumstances can cause havoc in the household and should be brought into the exit plan of what their responsibilities are.

5. Keeping the focus on the positive.

The exit strategy should ultimately be positive and not viewed as a *when-we-kick them-out* plan. Sometimes, parents feel guilty about setting some strict parameters when adult children move back home as they may think it is still their job to provide for their adult children. The key word, yet again, is *they are adults*. They are your equals and should be determined to make their way in life. Helping your adult children get back onto their feet is exactly what the focus should be on, and that is not an endless long-term situation. Creating a plan that will help your adult children feel good about themselves and achieve the ultimate goal of moving out and being stable once again is exactly what should be aimed for.

One of our adult children had a goal to save the deposit needed to enable them to purchase a house. We were aware of this right from the beginning and were invited to view some of the potential purchases as time went on. I love house-hunting, so I really enjoyed tagging along when I was asked.

Finally, the day came when an apartment went on the market that was selling via an auction, and they were able to place a bid. There was much celebration when their offer was accepted, and they were now proud owners of a home! The days and weeks leading up to the occupation date flew by with much excitement, particularly in those last few days of the countdown to the moving out and moving in day!

Another one of our adult children aimed to gain full-time employment following the collapse of the industry they had worked in due to the impact the COVID-19 pandemic had on the world. Subsequently, they gained a fantastic position in a prestigious workplace, and again we celebrated!

As the final week drew closer, there were undoubtedly many mixed emotions that surfaced. I was so proud that they had attained their goals, but I knew I would miss them terribly. Tears were shed privately, and I talked to friends who had been in the same situation and was comforted to know they had also experienced many different emotions in similar circumstances.

I think that it is a journey for parents right from the start of the cycle of building up and letting go, empowering and releasing; I just did not realize how significant the effect would be again when it happened now with them as adult children have already left the nest before. It does not get easier, but it does get more rewarding.

I know that your adult child will also be going through a myriad of emotions too, and acknowledging these emotions to each other is healthy.

Planning Life Post-Move-Out Day

Much will change in both the parent's and the adult child's life when they move out, apart from the obvious of not sharing a home anymore. Again, a flurry of emotions will surface for both of you at the beginning of this new stage.

Letting go and allowing your adult child to be independent is sometimes hard for some parents, particularly when they have been back at home for a long time. It is sometimes difficult to let go for many parents, and it is not an unusual emotion. Focus on believing in them and knowing that you have done everything possible to give them the tools to succeed.

Accept that even though you may feel sad, it is a happy time. Be grateful for the extra or bonus time you have had. Having a real-life glimpse into your child's life as an adult is not something all parents get a chance to experience. Hold onto those precious memories of the extra time you have had together. Give credit where credit is due, and do not hold back on compliments; instead, hold back on negative emotions. This time in your adult child's life is theirs, and you are an observer of them finding their way back into the big world.

As difficult as seeing them go, you know it has to happen at some stage so try to find another way of dealing with being sad that they are going. Think instead of a whole lot of new adventures ahead and how proud you are of them, instead of perhaps focusing on your feelings of sadness. Be positive and encourage them as much as you are doing it for yourself. Tell them they are ready to regain their independence and that they will achieve self-sufficiency with a life ahead that is full of purpose and adventure!

My reflections on all the good times kept me focused and helped me realize that my life would change again. I have always been a positive person who can see the cup as half full instead of half empty.

Acknowledge the benefits of having the house back to yourself. Some of these were being able to grab the remote to watch whatever you want when you want, cooking for fewer people, having more space in the house, and the ability to reconnect as a couple again. On the other hand, you may be so pleased as they head out the door, and no more plans are needed or structures to be agreed upon, you just dance madly around the house enjoying your newfound freedom!

Looking on the positive side, it was not as if I was lost with nothing to do since they moved out, as I always maintained my exercise schedule, time with God, and meeting with friends. It was important to me to keep living my life while they were living with us, and I am grateful I did this.

Ensure you create space while still maintaining contact with your adult children once they have moved out. They are embarking on a new journey and will be excited about this next stage, so, remember you are in the counselor role now. If they want advice, they know where to find you and will ask you if they need to.

In my situation, it was not long before we met at cafés, enjoyed shared stories, planned future family events, and shared life again.

10

RESOURCES FOR SETTING BOUNDARIES

The secret to getting ahead is getting started. The secret of getting started is breaking your complex overwhelming tasks into small manageable tasks and starting on the first one. –Mark Twain

When establishing your boundaries, some resistance might surface, particularly if it is something your adult child does not agree with. Being open to finding a compromise is the balance you are wanting to achieve. In this chapter, there are a few resources that you can choose to use to help guide you along the way. Reflecting on and clarifying your boundaries will help create a plan that can be agreed upon and minimize conflict.

These resources are suggested to supplement both the parent's and the adult child's plan to create an attainable living situation.

Some may view a contract with your adult child as being too heavy going or an unnecessary thing to do. Choosing whether or not to do this is entirely up to you, but the benefits of the contract will give some clarity and consistency to what you have agreed upon. Apart from this, a contract between you and your adult child may be the first one they have ever signed, so it is a life skill you are giving them as we all know how many agreements and documents we have to sign as adults! The sense of responsibility they will have for you is also not a bad thing.

If resentment crops up regarding your requirement, should you decide on having a contract, or comparisons about their friends not having to do the same, do not forget to stand your ground in instilling what is important to you. Your focus is to have clear guidelines and, in the end, create a happy household where everyone knows where they stand. Explaining to your adult child the benefit of learning about acceptance of consequences for their actions, both good and bad, is the cornerstone of growing up. Try to keep calm if the discussions about your need for a contract go pear-shaped, and explain the benefits are not only for you but also for them.

This agreement could include the expectations, goals, rules, or guidelines and what the consequences would be if they are not met. Compiling this contract together can be a beneficial tool for you and your adult child. Whatever you decide to be put in the contract will certainly depend on whether or not your adult child is working. If they have no means of income, then you will need to adjust your requirements to potentially include other things, such as responsibilities around the house.

The last word on the approach about needing a contract is to be sure to present this at the opportune time; ensuring you prepare them. Create a time and place where it can be presented and discussed without other distractions. This contract proposal is meant to come from a directive of caring for their well-being and yours too. It is about love and ensuring that they understand their opinion and input into this contract matters.

TEMPLATE OF A FAMILY CONTRACT

This template is just a suggestion and needs to work in your household and be reasonable to everyone involved. Please amend and craft as you see fit.

Family Contract	
This contract is between____ and ____	
It has been drawn up to outline the requirements and needs regarding living at ____ Address	
Start date_________________________	End date_________________________
If for whatever reason, the end date cannot be met and a new end date needs to be agreed upon, this contract must be renegotiated by: _________________________________ Date A new contract will be drawn up to be signed.	
Items:	
Accommodation: A weekly/fortnightly/monthly fee of _____________________ is to be paid by ___________________ If for whatever reason, this obligation cannot be met, advice thereof must be given by __________________________________ OR *It is agreed that for _____months, no accommodation contribution is required. Payments will commence on Date:* ____________________	
Household expenses: A weekly /fortnightly/monthly fee of ______________________ is to be paid commencing ____________________ This fee will cover contributions to the internet, power, gas and water and other utilities. Phone bills are at your own expense.	
Expectations and Requirements: 1. Family meetings are held weekly/fortnightly (circle as applicable). Designate the time: _______________________________ 2. Cooking duties will be split by agreement as agreed. If you are unable to adhere to your designated duty, then negotiate a swap with someone in the household. This should not become a habit and should only be used under exceptional circumstances or work commitments. 3. The communal areas, kitchen, lounge, and dining area must be kept neat at all times. 4. Shared bathrooms must be kept clean and tidy.	

<table>
<tr><td>

5. Everyone is responsible for their laundry. No wet laundry is to be visible in internal communal areas.
6. No smoking or use of drugs is permitted in the house.
7. Excessive alcohol consumption is discouraged.
8. If a vehicle is to be borrowed, it must be returned clean and with the same fuel tank level it was when borrowed.
9. Additional responsibilities may include lawns/gardening/rubbish disposal (circle as applicable). Substitute or add others as required.
10. Visitors are welcome – it is appreciated if this is communicated to other members of the household. Use of communal areas when having visitors must be respectful to other household members.
11. Communication about lateness for meals or not coming home is appreciated.

</td></tr>
<tr><td>

Home office expenses (if applicable):

1. For the first ______ month/s, no contribution is required. Thereafter, depending on the usage of printers and paper, etc., an agreement on a contribution will be made upon discussion.
2. The use of the office is a privilege and space will be provided for you to continue your remote work.
3. The office will not be available to you between the hours of ______ and ______ Any remote work you need to complete during these times will have to be done in your own space.

</td></tr>
<tr><td>

Breach:

1. If the above requirements are in breach under any circumstances, a written warning will be presented. An opportunity to address this written warning will be available at our required family meetings. Three warnings will result in the termination of this contract.

</td></tr>
<tr><td>Signed
____
Name
______________________________ Date______________________________</td></tr>
<tr><td>Signed
____
Name
______________________________ Date______________________________</td></tr>
<tr><td>Signed
____
Name
______________________________ Date______________________________</td></tr>
</table>

HELPING PLANNING BUDGETS

As your adult child has come home for assistance in getting themselves back on their feet, it could be helpful to guide them in helping plan a budget both for the short-term and the long-term.

Depending on your financial circumstances, perhaps the rental you have suggested could be split into two where one half is saved for them. This could be discussed with them or you could save it quietly and present them with a nest egg when they move out.

Of critical importance is to be clear about what you can offer financially, if anything. If you cannot, that is okay. What is important is to be clear about it. If you are in a position to help them financially, clarify the terms and the period you can assist so that they, in turn, have time to prepare themselves for taking on those expenses. If you promise financial help with no clear guidelines, this could create problems down the line.

Helping your adult children build a good credit record is invaluable support. So, they could potentially have access to applying for future loans for a home or vehicle when they are in a sound financial position to do so. Getting into debt is not the objective here; it is creating a good credit record.

The integral part of budgeting for needs and not wants is the tricky part. Suggesting that they list the needs and wants in two columns on a piece of paper can give them a good visual of the differences.

Using technology to track their expenses is also a great idea or they can create a spreadsheet and list their income and expenses and see where their shortfall is they have to make up. Instilling saving something every single month, no matter how little, is a fantastic habit to have. This can be motivated by explaining that saving is investing in their future and not just to have extra spending money.

Talk about creating nest eggs and how to be wise about these numerous get-rich-quick scams. Mention how starting now with putting money away gives them a massive head start in securing their future.

Some adult children may be secretive about sharing their financial situation with you, and it may be from embarrassment or just that they want privacy. Encouraging them to share this with you might be a hard task but persevere from an angle of support and experience. And yes, as always, from love for them.

SCHEDULING PERSONAL BOUNDARIES AND COMMUNAL TIME

Sharing a home can be tricky! Steps to make it a bit easier are to be sure you are clear with the boundaries you require to keep your sanity intact.

1. Do not be vague. Say to your adult child that you think it might not be great if they smoked inside, but if they did it only a few times it would be okay. This is a sure way of sending confusing information. Be clear. Either no smoking inside or smoke inside.
2. Housework schedules can be drafted on a whiteboard, showing who has what responsibility that week so it is understood. This might sound a little administrative, but in the end, it will help clarify who was meant to do what.
3. Accountability is so important for growth. Even if you come up with the consequences of actions not followed through with your adult child, this can also be helpful as they would feel part of creating the solutions and requirements instead of just being told what to do.
4. Clarify the expectations and conditions of house guests. This is a personal thing and will depend on many factors. Talk about it with each other and come to an agreement that will satisfy everyone.
5. Set times for family time and communicate the importance of finding time to connect and discuss things together at a certain time and place. Make time for fun and connect with each other. Nurture the special relationship you are creating with your adult child.

6. Agree on private space for yourselves and them and acknowledge the respect and need for privacy as adults.
7. Do not compare your situation to other families as their circumstances or personalities are different. Focus on what is best for your family.
8. Learn to listen when communicating and resist the urge to respond immediately, particularly if it is something you do not agree with.
9. Talk about shared responsibilities whether they are physical or monetary contributions.
10. Share your life experiences without focusing on the in-my-day scenario. You both are from different generations and things are definitely different. Talk about it and find the comparative differences and similarities where perhaps a solution can be found for a problem raised.

COPING MECHANISMS WHEN THINGS GET TOUGH

Having some mechanisms to use to help you cope with tough situations is good preparation. Never be afraid to ask for help if you feel you are not coping. There are many associations available to help you if you do not have a support structure.

If you have close friends who you can trust and are able to blow off some steam with or just need to talk it out without even wanting or needing a solution, you are fortunate. Use these avenues to gain some perspective and support that you might need.

Patience is most often the crux of dealing with challenging situations. Perhaps some of the expectations you have of your adult child are too much for them to deal with and they are not coping. Having the literal open-door policy with your adult children will help if they feel the need to approach you but not all households operate like this. Perhaps some extenuating circumstances are bothering them and might make them feel inadequate, or they are a big disappointment to you if they cannot perform as you might have expected. This may be so far from what you are actually wanting, but if they are feeling like this, then you need to be aware of it.

Earlier in the book, it was proposed to have regular family meetings. These times together are very important for identifying any underlying issues, and the tools suggested below will hopefully help ease the process forward rather than backward. Keep the communication at these meetings open and flowing with no harsh words or judgment of one another. Creating a safe platform to be able to speak without attacking or accusing one another is what you want to have—even if this means implementing a system of a *talking stick* if the tendency is to speak over one another and deal with constant interruptions. Just because you are the parents does not give you free rein to overrule and talk over your adult children, and the same goes for them. Reverting to childish behavior and stomping off to have a good sulk is not helpful at all. There are other ways to leave a confrontational environment with tact and maintain respect for one another.

More often, the boundaries become an issue for adult children as they do not want to be treated like a child and be told what to do. Keeping your discussion open about these boundaries and how they can be improved will help avoid serious confrontations.

Stress and Conflict Management Tools

- Do your utmost to avoid avoidance.

Sometimes, it is easier just to avoid conflict and hope that it goes away. It may very well go away for a time, but often when issues are not resolved properly, they will most certainly surface again. Every time they surface, they are more likely to be more difficult to deal with. Be conscious of facing up to difficult issues and do your utmost to deal with them in a way that is kind and productive.

- Bringing competitiveness into a situation is bad news.

Even small comparisons about other adult children or other parents can raise defensiveness, and then the walls are up and difficult to break down. Nobody likes to be compared negatively to another. Focus on your situation and try not to make comparisons. There is no harm in setting goals to achieve that others have reached, but the realization that the paths followed for you to get there may be different.

- Being the one to compromise in various situations.

Avoid being the one who consistently gives in and vice versa, do not be the dogmatic one who refuses to try to find a balanced solution and is steadfast in only seeing things their way. Depending on the circumstances, this sometimes is necessary when breaking laws and so on, but this is not applicable regarding this point raised now. It is about being able to take both sides of a story and listening and speaking to each other civilly about your differences to find a way that is an equal compromise. A friend gave me some great advice: "Always be the first to apologize and take the moral high ground. Be humble and this will gain you respect."

- Using collaboration to reach an agreement.

When a stressful situation has evolved, everyone is affected, not just you. Using this as a positive instead of a negative to reach a resolution is possible. Sometimes, we are so stuck in our misery about some circumstances that are making life difficult that we do not realize that those closest to us are feeling the same way. It is kind of finding sense in the madness if you like! Talking, listening, and considering each other when you have these regular meetings that are integral to the pursuit of positivity, will bring this to light if you allow it.

CONCLUSION

Excellence is never an accident. It is always the result of high intention, sincere effort, and intelligent execution; it represents the wise choice of many alternatives-choice, not chance determines your destiny. –Aristotle

This time in your life may be a trying one for everyone that is involved in it, but it seriously does not have to be. Take a moment to acknowledge the opportunity you have been presented with to spend some time with your adult child. This is not available for all parents as some children fly the coop early and sometimes have very little to do with their parents' lives. Looking at a situation that could be a difficult one and adjusting your perspective by reframing it in a positive light will affect the most significant change. Be grateful that your adult children love and trust you enough to want to come home again.

This process might not be easy for them either, as many teenagers yearn to be adults and move out as soon as they can. They are desperate to make their own choices and live their own way, and now that has changed for them and they are back where they started. Being mindful of the emotional turmoil that they are experiencing instead of just looking at it negatively that they did not make it out in the big world, is crucial in establishing your common ground together as adults. In the same way, your adult child needs to acknowledge the opportunity given to them to take a bit more time to establish themselves when they should be out of the home by that stage.

Some guidelines in this book have been offered to you to implement in a way that suits your household. What is fundamental in making it a smooth process is to be sure to support yourself and your needs during this time. It is hard for some parents to learn how to switch off the parental instinct that we have had for all our children's lives. This is not the time to be focused purely on your adult child's needs but yours too.

The various strategies that have been presented can be honed to suit your needs but what is vital is not to omit a structure to work with. This does not mean that you do not have to be flexible with what has been decided upon, but be aware of not compromising yourself and your spouse, whether it is intentional or unintentional.

Welcoming your adult child back into your home is a common phenomenon all over the world, particularly post-pandemic, where many lives remain shattered. You are not alone in this situation, and many of us need help to get ourselves back together and back on track. Being in the position to help and support your adult child through a difficult patch they are going through is a gift that they should value.

KEY LESSONS

Let us restate the key points in this book that are the most influential in this boomerang process.

1. The initial request and your reaction to it must be monitored.

Never has there been a time to gauge your reaction to one of the most important people in your life. Keeping in touch with your adult children but still allowing them the freedom to live their lives can give you a head start just in case this request is imminent.

2. Communication is more than just talking.

Slow it down, listen more, and you will hear what needs to be communicated. Shutting off those responses that shout in your head when someone is talking to you takes practice. Remember that if you are a good listener, your adult children will keep communicating with you.

3. Create boundaries and non-negotiables together.

Having clear boundaries in place and being flexible with your ideas of what they will be will help with those non-negotiables you would not want to be changed.

4. Identify your common ground with each other.

Finding this common ground with your adult child is such a lovely and welcome surprise to explore together. It could also be a time to learn new things about each other and explore endless possibilities.

5. Be realistic about the expectations of each other and what the ultimate goals are.

Remember that expectations are not set, and much will depend on what is going on inside your head. Talking about your expectations and sharing your inner thoughts helps you to be realistic about expectations. Revisit your goals and do not be too harsh with setting realistic time frames, etc.

6. Establish this new adult-adult relationship with your child.

Stepping into the shoes and becoming a parent of adult children is as if a new world has opened up. You know these people intimately, yet they are now different. The greatest joy is seeing your children become independent adults. Sharing a glimpse of their step into adulthood is a blessing, and it is to be cherished.

7. Find your peace and maintain your sanity.

Sometimes it won't be easy and will challenge everyone in the household because it is different, and you are all adults now. Change is inevitable. Having a way to step away from negativity and find your inner calm to deal with it productively is an absolute must.

8. The absolute joy it is to have this time with your adult child and to be able to explore your newfound relationship together.

Not all parents have this opportunity with their adult children as it is different when they live in their own homes. Having this time is precious and must be treasured. Do not sweat the small stuff and make the moments with each other count.

9. Establish and agree on the exit plan for when they move out.

Clarifying this ahead of time is very important so everyone in the household knows where they stand. Extenuating circumstances can arise and if you have a structure in place that can be adapted, it will make everything a lot easier and result in less stress.

10. Use the resources available to support this process.

The resources offered in this book are to give you the information and tools to assist in helping set a framework for this new relationship living together as adults.

THE LAST WORD

This book has been a labor of love with the intention of sharing what has been experienced personally and in our close friends' lives who have been in a similar situation. It is understood that there will be varying differences in circumstances in your home and the methods and advice included in the book have been considered carefully to be able to be adapted. Using this information offered to you and adjusting it to your life will be beneficial to you and your family.

It is also intended to enable the ability to move forward into the future together with your adult child with stability, support, and keeping the love alive you have for each other. I hope this book helps you to minimize conflicts and maximize opportunities to strengthen your family bonds. Our experience living together again as a family of adults was challenging but enlightening and fulfilling.

"There is no passion to be found playing small, in settling for a life that is less than the one you are capable of living" (Nelson Mandela, as cited in AZ Quotes, n.d.-h).

REFERENCES

Abraham, K., & Studaker-Cordner, M. (2022). *6 steps to help your child move out*. Empowering Parents. https://www.empoweringparents.com/article/failure-to-launch-part-3-six-steps-to-help-your-adult-child-move-out/

AZ Quotes. (n.d.-a). *A quote by Aristotle*. https://www.azquotes.com/author/524-Aristotle

AZ Quotes. (n.d.-b). *A quote by Brad Henry*. https://www.azquotes.com/author/6571-Brad_Henry

AZ Quotes. (n.d.-c). *A quote by Eva Burrows*. https://www.azquotes.com/quote/1393507

AZ Quotes. (n.d.-d). *A quote by Mark Twain*. https://www.azquotes.com/quote/399388

AZ Quotes. (n.d.-e). *A quote by Maya Angelou*. https://www.azquotes.com/author/440-Maya_Angelou

AZ Quotes. (n.d.-f). *A quote by Michael Shurtleff*. https://www.azquotes.com/author/21779-Michael_Shurtleff

AZ Quotes. (n.d.-g). *A quote by Mitch Albom*. https://www.azquotes.com/author/195-Mitch_Albom

AZ Quotes. (n.d.-h). *A quote by Nelson Mandela*. https://www.azquotes.com/quote/185314

AZ Quotes. (n.d.-i). *A quote by Spike Milligan*. https://www.azquotes.com/quote/564542

AZ Quotes. (n.d.-j). *A quote by Tony Robbins*. https://www.azquotes.com/author/12429-Tony_Robbins

AZ Quotes. (n.d.-k). *A quote by Mark Victor Hansen*. https://www.azquotes.com/quote/368977

Butler, P. (2020, October 18). *"Boomerang" trend of young adults living with parents is rising – study*. The Guardian. https://www.theguardian.com/society/2020/oct/18/boomerang-trend-of-young-adults-living-with-parents-is-rising-study

Cambridge Dictionary. (2022, July 13). *Snowflake generation*. https://dictionary.cambridge.org/dictionary/english/snowflake-generation

Carrane, L. (2015, November 27). *7 tips for when your young adult children move back home*. Psych Central. https://psychcentral.com/blog/7-tips-for-when-your-young-adult-children-move-back-home#5

Clark, D. (2022, April 28). *Young adults living with parents UK 2020*. Statista. https://www.statista.com/statistics/285339/percentage-of-young-adults-living-with-parents-uk/

Conversation, A. T. (2020, July 7). *Brace yourself: Over 50% of young Australian adults still live with their parents*. Mumlyfe. https://mumlyfe.com.au/still-live-with-parents/

Dastoor, C. (2021, March 17). *"Boomerang generation" bounces out*. Money Management. https://www.moneymanagement.com.au/news/financial-planning/boomerang-generation-bounces-out

Hess, A. J. (2022, January 10). *How "boomerang kids" who moved back home show the unequal economic effects of the pandemic*. CNBC. https://www.cnbc.com/2022/01/10/young-adults-with-rich-parents-are-more-likely-to-boomerang-back-home.html

Hayes, A. (2022, March 13). *Boomerang children*. Investopedia. https://www.investopedia.com/terms/b/boomerangs.asp

Hostetler, B. (2007, January 1). *The four phases of parenthood*. Focus on the Family. https://www.focusonthefamily.com/parenting/the-four-phases-of-parenthood/

Kennedy, L. P., & Farrell, P. A. (2019). *What to do when adult children want to move back in*. WebMD. https://www.webmd.com/parenting/features/adult-children-move-back-in

Lehman, J. (2022). *Living agreement with adult children.* Empowering Parents. https://www.empoweringparents.com/article/rules-boundaries-and-older-children-part-iii-is-it-ever-too-late-to-set-up-a-living-agreement/

Leidy, L. (2021, July 6). *5 financial steps Gen Z should be taking now*. GOBankingRates. https://www.gobankingrates.com/money/financial-planning/financial-steps-gen-z-should-be-taking-now/

Lisa, A. (2021, September 15). *The pros and cons of living at home vs. moving out*. Yahoo Finance. https://finance.yahoo.com/news/pros-cons-living-home-vs-150111133.html

McCarthy, K. (2021, August 30). *Tips for when adult children move back home*. LoveToKnow. https://family.lovetoknow.com/about-family-values/tips-when-adult-children-move-back-home

McCarthy, K. (n.d.). *Example contract for an adult child living at home*. LoveToKnow. https://family.lovetoknow.com/parenting-tips-strategies-modern-world/example-contract-adult-child-living-at-home

Newport Institute. (2021, March 25). *Tips for families with young adults moving back home*. https://www.newportinstitute.com/resources/co-occurring-disorders/moving-back-home/

Obenschain, C. (2011, May 4). *5 tips for dealing with an adult child moving home*. HowStuffWorks. https://lifestyle.howstuffworks.com/family/parenting/parenting-tips/5-tips-for-dealing-with-adult-child-moving-home.htm

PassItOn. (n.d.). *A quote by George Washington Carver*. https://www.passiton.com/common-ground

Peng, T. (2008, December 17). *How to cope when your adult kids move back home.* Newsweek. https://www.newsweek.com/how-cope-when-your-adult-kids-move-back-home-83475

Pincus, D. (2022). *9 rules for your child living at home.* Empowering Parents. https://www.empoweringparents.com/article/adult-children-living-at-home-part-ii-9-rules-to-help-you-maintain-sanity/

Poole, S. (2020, August 10). *Remember these 7 things as your young adults move out for good.* Grown and Flown. https://grownandflown.com/7-tips-parents-young-adults-move-out-for-good/

Raypole, C. (2020, February 11). *Interpersonal conflict: What it is and how to resolve it.* Healthline. https://www.healthline.com/health/interpersonal-conflict#takeaway

The Holy Bible, New International Version. (2011). Biblica. https://www.biblica.-com/online-bible/ (Original work published in 1973)

Wagner, B. (2021, December 23). *Fact check: 47% of American young adults currently live with their parents.* USA TODAY. https://www.usatoday.com/story/news/factcheck/2021/12/23/fact-check-47-american-young-adults-live-their-parents/8672598002/

Yu, A. (2022). *The adult "boomerang kids" moving home to their parents.* BBC. https://www.bbc.com/worklife/article/20220208-the-adult-boomerang-kids-moving-home-to-their-parents

ABOUT THE AUTHOR

Victoria Lynch, who lives in beautiful New Zealand, is the loving wife of a total geek who is an information technology enthusiast. She is blessed to be a mother to two adult children, stepmother to another two adult children, and nana to three grandchildren. She makes up the nucleus of the family. Not forgetting Max, the one-eyed cat who rules the roost above everyone!

An avid writer, she has to have a cup of coffee in hand to keep the cogs turning, and when not writing, she spends her time walking, practicing yoga, making lists, or enjoying the freedom of exploring nature. She has had a diverse career, from studying animal husbandry and applied management to Christian leadership, and tertiary education, before plunging into being a writer.

Gregarious and optimistic are two words to describe Victoria, who has the incredible capacity to mentor and motivate others to find a better version of themselves.

Printed in Great Britain
by Amazon